SISTER OF MY FRIEND

Levi Orion

1

Cedric von Hohenburg, an eighteen-year-old student from Munich, was allowed to go on vacation with the family of his best friend Harry.

For almost three months he had been begging his parents to let him go with them. After a three-hour drive, they reached the Zillertal in Austria.

For Cedric, the ride flew by as he sat snuggled up against Harry's sister in the back seat of the car. Slender Anna had to sit in the middle, which she wasn't thrilled about.

The Mayrhofen campsite is in a quiet, sunny location on the northern edge of the small town, right on the edge of the forest. The first night had been wonderful.

Cedric had never slept in a tent before. Most of the time he had looked at the clear starry sky. He hadn't even shown any interest in the various sex magazines that Harry wanted to show him. He didn't fall asleep until morning. Today they had spent almost exclusively hiking through the mountains of the Zillertal. The landscape was fantastically beautiful, the weather sunny and warm.

Marcel Plessen, Harry's father, was an experienced mountaineer and could tell a lot about nature.

Cedric was completely happy.

Until now he had only known about campfires and tent camps from books. He had always dreamed of experiencing something like this himself.

In the evening they heated up the grill.

Carolin Plessen, Harry's mother, took care of the food.

It was so warm that everyone wore only light clothing. So he could watch Anna well. Harry's twenty-one-year-old sister wore her long, blue-black hair in a ponytail. The tight t-shirt gave a hint of her firm breasts.

But Carolin, the mother of the round, also had a lot to offer. She was always funny and cheerful, joking with everyone and having fun teasing everyone. Her T-shirt suggested an even larger bust size. Carolin also had black hair and a very good figure for her thirty-nine years.

Harry nudged Cedric with a grin.

"So what do you think of my sister's tits?" he whispered.

"They're kind of great," Cedric replied, slightly embarrassed. He didn't want to tell his best friend that he was secretly in love with Anna.

After dinner, Carolin suggested grilling some bananas on what was left of the embers. Just before the fruit was ready, the weather changed. This happened in the mountains within a few minutes.

It was just a warm midsummer evening, then the sky darkened and a thunderstorm approached. They rushed to stow the equipment in the tents. Before the rain started, they fled to their tents.

Harry's parents slept in a large tent that offered enough space for luggage and equipment. Harry and Cedric lived in a much smaller tent. Anna insisted on having her own place to sleep, so she slept in a tiny tent that only fit one person.

Harry had often experienced rain while camping. His parents have been choosing this type of vacation for years. He crawled into his sleeping bag and flipped through his porn collection.

Despite the violent thunderstorm, Harry quickly fell asleep. Cedric, on the other hand, listened to the sound of the drops and the song of the wind. He kept thinking about Anna. He had dreamed of Harry's sister for a long time.

She was his secret love, his secret jerk off template.

Not even Harry knew about it.

Anna was almost as tall as him. He was particularly taken with her long, blue-black hair. When she wore it open, it hung to her hips. The color changed from a blue-black to a jet-black depending on the sunlight. Cedric knew every shade of color.

Something else fascinated him about Anna. It was her long legs that ended in a heart-shaped bottom. Unconsciously he grabbed his best piece when he thought about Anna and massaged it. He began to dream, the main role was played by his friend's older sister, as always.

A noise tore him out of his fantasies!

The tent was opened from the outside. Cedric hastily reached for the flashlight while at the same time pulling up his trousers, which was not so easy in the sleeping bag. In the dim light he saw Anna crawling into the tent with her sleeping bag.

“Hello Cedy, my tent is leaking. How are you all doing?"

"I think we're all right."

"Harry is probably asleep as usual, not even a storm can stop him. Can I lie down with you? I don't want to go to my parents' main tent."

"Yeah, sure."

Cedric scooted to the side as far as he could. Anna put her sleeping bag next to him and crawled inside. He turned off the flashlight again.

"Are you cold too?" she whispered softly.

"No, I'm warm."

"That's the advantage of young men, they're hot all the time."

She chuckled softly at her own sentence.

"I'm shivering."

"If you had a few more pounds, you wouldn't be cold," Cedric replied quietly.

"Then there wouldn't be so many men whistling at me!"

Cedric could almost see her mischievous grin. As always, she had managed that he couldn't come up with a funny reply. He felt shy around her, like a pubescent teenager.

Nothing stirred for a long time.

He thought he only heard the chattering of her teeth occasionally.

"I'm so cold. May I warm up with you?"

Cedric froze. What did she want?

"Uhhh... what do you mean?"

He turned on his side to make more room for Anna's sleeping bag. But she didn't scoot closer with her sleeping bag. He froze when he heard her unzip her sleeping bag. Then the noise again. But this time it was the zip from his own sleeping bag. She climbed over to him and made herself comfortable next to him. She quickly closed the zip again.

A little later he felt her cold feet. They were like lumps of ice.

"Hm, it's really nice and warm where you live."

She turned onto her side and hugged him tightly. Cedric didn't dare to move. He lay there paralyzed. It was slowly getting warmer in the sleeping bag.

"Cedy, you're a good stove. I'm already much warmer."

He sniffed, smelled her perfume, turned to her and placed his hand on her hip. Anna immediately pressed herself against him. She took his hand and placed it on her stomach. His thumb rested just below her breast.

That touch increased his confusion and unnerved his pants. Slowly but inexorably his erection increased. He felt that he had to do something soon. His member had gotten lost in his underpants, was bent and was beginning to hurt.

Anna, on the other hand, seemed to welcome the growth in his pants. She pressed her butt tighter and harder against him. Cedric was uncomfortable with this, he was shy and nervous. When, after a few contortions, he had finally freed his member from the forced situation, he breathed a sigh of relief and leaned against Anna again.

"Cedy, that feels good," she whispered.

He thought about what to say, but again he couldn't think of anything.

Anna, on the other hand, seemed too comfortable. She rubbed her buttocks against his member more and more firmly. She took his hand and placed it on her breast. He was only too happy to grab it.

While he shyly felt the flesh of her bust, she looked for a way into his pants with her hand.

"Cedy, that's a nice surprise. I didn't expect you to be so big and firm."

"Stop with the cedy. It sounds like a stuffed animal, so childish."

"Oh go, the name suits you. I think the acronym is cute."

He couldn't believe his ears. What did she say?

Did you think his name was cute?

His pulse quickened.

While he was still thinking about it, his fingers did their thing, examining her breasts. She didn't appear to be wearing a bra under her tracksuit top.

Carefully he looked for the zipper to open the jacket. After a long search he finally found it. He slowly pulled it, but nothing moved. Only with their help was it possible to open the jacket.

As he explored the soft curves, Anna was more interested in the hardness of his cock.

She massaged him harder and harder!

Cedric took that as approval to further his own explorations. Anna definitely had a lot more breasts than he had ever laid hands on. What he liked was not only the size, but also the firmness, like that of an athlete. She had round yet comfortably soft breasts.

Suddenly she stopped his groping fingers.

"Slow and softer. The bosom has to last longer. Don't crush it the first time."

She showed him how she imagined it.

Relief spread over him as she let go of his member. He knew from his numerous self-experiments that he was already close to cumming. He breathed a sigh of relief when his excitement had subsided a little.

Anna was a good teacher.

Together with her fingers, he quickly learned how to handle her breasts. Suddenly he felt a small but all the harder structure between his fingers. Puzzled, his fingers examined the novelty. Anna moans softly as he rolls her aroused nipples between his fingers. But the biggest surprise was yet to come.

"I think I have to take off my jacket. I'm so warm already."

Anna suddenly began to undress!

Which was not so easy in the tight sleeping bag. When she finally made it, she turned to Cedric.

"Would you like to keep playing with my boobs? It wasn't bad what you did there before. But you mustn't get rough again."

Cedric couldn't believe it!

His dream came true!

Anna wanted him to play with her bare breasts.

He carefully began to caress her firm curves. She seemed to agree with his timid attempts. Slowly he became bolder and dared to grab a little harder. When he felt her nipples getting hard again, he fulfilled another dream.

He bent his head down and licked her nipples with the tip of his tongue.

"You're doing wonderfully, Cedy, you're a real expert."

Sudden lightning and loud thunder interrupted his game as Harry began to toss and turn in his sleep. He didn't wake up, just rolled over a few times, then seemed to be sound asleep again.

Cedric just started stroking her breasts again when they heard their parents' voices.

"Anna? Where are you?" her father called.

"I'm here with Harry and Cedric. It rains into my stupid tent. The fabric has leaked."

"Are you okay?" asked Carolin, her mother.

"Yes, of course. Everything OK. My sleeping bag stayed dry. It's a little tight, but it's okay."

"Okay, good night then. We'll have a look at your tent tomorrow," her father said.

Cedric took a deep breath. He was already afraid that her parents would look into the tent and find them together in a sleeping bag.

"Cedylein, don't you want to take off your shirt too?" Anna brought him back to the present.

"Uhh... do you really mean... uhh... I..."

"Come on, it's so warm in here."

Obediently but uncertainly, he began to remove his shirt.

Anna seemed to read his reaction correctly.

"Cedy, have you ever?"

"What... uhh... do you mean?"

"Sex."

"Yes... no... not really."

"Do you like?"

"With you?" he stammered, completely insecure.

"Is there another woman present?"

"No."

"So? Do you feel like?"

"Yes...uh...but I don't know...uh."

Anna gently stroked his cheek.

"Don't worry, I'll show you how to do it."

Cedric swallowed. He had wanted to sleep with a woman for so long. And now this! The dream of his sleepless nights, his secret goddess herself, offered to sleep with him.

But only a few inches away was sleeping his best friend, who could wake up at any moment. In addition, her parents slept in the tent next door. And he didn't even have a condom with him. Never in his life would he have thought he would need it here.

Anna seemed to be able to read his mind.

"Don't get nervous. Once Harry falls asleep, nothing will wake him up that easily. My parents are busy themselves, they fuck every night on vacation. Do you have a condom?"

"No...uh...I didn't think I'd be sleeping with a woman here on vacation. Actually, I rather thought that a girl would never sleep with me."

"It doesn't matter! I brought one from my tent."

"How come?"

"I wanted you."

Again he got no answer. Her closeness and directness left him speechless. She rummaged in her pants and soon found what she was looking for.

"Relax yourself."

Cedric took a deep breath and let it out again.

How should he relax in this situation?

Anna took the condom out of the packaging and slipped it over his hard penis.

"Actually, we don't need a condom. I'm on the pill, but that way we won't stain your sleeping bag."

Skillfully she checked the fit of the condom. That touch almost made him come. His sperm was already in front of his glans, ready for freedom. Anna let him go just in time.

She snuggled up to him and started kissing him. Timidly he returned her touch. Her lips were warm and soft. There was nothing hesitant or uncertain about it. She knew what she wanted. Slowly but surely he returned her kiss. He parted his lips and tentatively touched the tip of his tongue to her mouth.

How good it tastes, how great it smells.

His heart was racing.

She pressed herself against him and rubbed her slim body against him. When he wanted to lie down on her, she refused.

"Take your time. I'm not running away."

Wait, how should he wait?

His dream just came true!

But Anna knew how to stop him. She kissed and caressed him. Then she guided his hand between her legs. Curious, his fingers touched her pubic hair.

Anna shivered at his touch and moaned softly.

Her intimate hair was trimmed to a maximum of one centimeter. With his fingertips he could feel that she was completely shaved at the edge and around her labia. There appeared to be only a short triangle.

Anna moaned softly when his finger entered her vagina for the first time, rather unintentionally.

"You're doing well, Cedylein."

She put her hand on his and pressed his finger deep inside her.

"Move your finger gently inside me," she instructed.

He didn't need to be told twice. He shoved his middle finger deep into her wet cunt, kept still, twisted it a little, then pulled it out again to penetrate again.

Anna was breathing faster and faster. She pressed her face against his shoulder to keep from moaning too loud.

"Cedy, now I want to feel something different inside me."

She pulled his finger out of its sheath and climbed onto him.

The tightness of the sleeping bag pressed them tightly together. Cedric cupped her firm breasts with both hands. This was better than he had imagined in his wildest dreams.

She moved her slender body and pressed herself firmly against his member. And before he knew it, she had reached her goal.

Slowly his stiff penis penetrated her vagina!

Cedric was completely overwhelmed by this feeling. He knew there was no stopping him now. He nudged his pelvis hard against her body a few times.

After a few seconds he exploded moaning loudly while continuing to massage her breasts. Anna put her hand over his mouth, muffling his outburst.

"Cedy! Cedy! You're one of the very fast troops."

Cedric flinched, taking his hands off her bosom when he heard that. Deep down, he wished he had never let her in his sleeping bag. He felt a deep sadness, he thought he had failed completely. Tears formed in his eyes.

Anna instinctively realized that she had made a mistake. She leaned forward and kissed him gently on the mouth. At the same time she began to move her pelvis again. She was still holding his cock in her sheath.

"Ceddy, I'm sorry. i didn't mean to hurt you It was stupid what I said. I'm really sorry. And what's more, where you came so beautifully."

She kissed him again without stopping her pelvis movement for even a second.

Tears ran down Cedric's cheeks. His worst nightmare had come true. He had come too soon and had disappointed her.

Anna lay down next to him and tried to comfort him. He turned his back on her and sobbed. She stroked him gently. But it took a long time for him to overcome this disappointment.

"Come face me again," she beckoned.

He turned around hesitantly.

"I was stupid what I said. I'm really sorry."

She kissed him softly, tenderly and full of feeling. Cedric felt himself relax. Anna's fingers had found their way to his member.

"I think we should get a new condom."

She gently pulled the rubber off his penis. With her panties she wiped his sperm away.

She kissed him and stroked his cock with her fingernails. It felt amazing!

To his amazement he got an erection again. Anna immediately rolled a new condom over his hard penis.

She didn't give him time for further considerations, climbed onto him again. He immediately grabbed her breasts again.

"Do you like my boobs?"

"Yes, he is beautiful, almost as beautiful as you."

Did he really say that?

He felt himself blush with embarrassment. Luckily she couldn't see that in the darkness of the tent.

Anna leaned towards him and kissed him. She enjoyed his compliment. It sounded so different than what she knew. Kind of honest. The compliments of late had all had one purpose, to get her into bed.

Cedric presses against her and after a few attempts his member penetrated her vagina again.

"Cedric?"

"Yes Anna?"

"Don't tense up unnecessarily. If you come, then you come. As simple as that."

"And you?"

"Do not worry. I'll get my money's worth. Just keep being such a dear Cedylein."

After another kiss, she sat up and began to move. She accompanied each of her pelvic movements with a firm grip on his member.

It didn't take long and Cedric moaned louder and louder. Anna put a hand over his mouth to muffle his noises. Her ring finger slipped into his mouth. He immediately started sucking her finger. suck. Surprised, Anna noticed that she was incredibly aroused.

He cupped her firm buttocks in his hands. He massaged her, pressed, rubbed and found her rosette with his fingertips.

Anna hoped it would stay that way, as she found anal stimulation unexciting. But today it felt completely different!

Cedric made no attempt to insert his finger into her. His massage was so arousing that she too had problems not getting loud. Again and again he pressed his finger firmly against her sphincter, but he did nothing more.

He moved more and more violently under her. Anna was looking forward to his next ejaculation. She loved it when she could feel the hot reward for her efforts. But this time it should be different.

Cedric's fingers excited her in a way she had never seen before.

His fingers slid faster and more excitedly over her back entrance.

Suddenly she is overwhelmed by a tremendous orgasm!

She supported herself on his chest and rode wildly on his huge cock. The excitement made her forget everything. She only felt the approaching orgasm. Anna gasped and moaned.

Cedric was still trapped by his fear of disappointing the woman of his dreams. He wanted to restrain himself, but his arousal increased with every movement.

He pushed his pelvis against her abdomen more and more violently, while his fingers continued to slide over her rosette. Anna leaned back, her hands wrapped around her breasts, letting the violent thrusts carry her. Without warning, his finger penetrated her sphincter.

Anna gasped in shock.

Harry tossed and turned restlessly in his sleep. The loud noises in the tent disturbed his sleep. Just as he woke up, Anna collapsed.

She fell onto Cedric and kissed him hard.

She had never experienced such a violent orgasm!

Cedric was out of his mind. He pushed his pelvis against her abdomen more and more violently, while their tongues performed a wild dance.

Harry woke up briefly.

He smelled Anna's perfume. He greedily sucked in the scent deeply, but then turned back onto the other side and leaned in again.

He didn't notice what was happening in the tent, just as the two didn't notice that Harry had woken up briefly.

Cedric didn't notice her orgasm. He was too busy with his own feelings. Only when he had discharged himself with violent moans did he notice that Anna was lying on him, stunned.

"Cedy! Cedy! That was great," she whispered in his ear, gently nibbling on his earlobe.

Although he enjoyed the feeling, it soon became too heavy for him. Anna lay down next to him and snuggled into the crook of his arm.

"I'm going to crawl back into my sleeping bag and sleep for a few more hours. Not much is left of the night. He was beautiful, Cedy. If you want, we'll do it again soon. Do you like?

"Yes... sure... I can't dream of anything nicer."

"Give me another kiss," she demanded tenderly.

A hinted kiss turned into a loving cuddle. He was reluctant to let his goddess go. But it was better this way. What would happen if Harry found them together in their sleeping bags tomorrow? They quickly got dressed again. Everyone lay in their sleeping bags.

Cedric turned to the tent wall and once again enjoyed the memory of the evening. Anna's perfume was hanging in the sleeping bag, he smelled it with pleasure.

"Sleep well, my cedyle."

"Good night Anna."

He was so exhausted that he soon fell asleep. Anna lay motionless in her sleeping bag and listened to her breathing. When she was sure that Cedric had fallen asleep, she unbuttoned her jeans and started stroking her short pubic hair.

She thought about the evening.

She had noticed all evening that Cedric had been secretly watching her. She had liked her brother's shy boyfriend from the start. Of course he was too young for her and she had never thought about sleeping with him. But today she just felt like it.

And Cedric was just a sweet boy. He was slim with a muscular, athletic body and dark brown hair. From the start she found his bright green eyes most interesting. They radiated passion, feeling and warmth.

Too bad he was only eighteen. At twenty-one, there was no way she could get involved with a youngster like that.

As she pondered, she kept stroking herself. Now she dipped a finger into her crack. Her excitement increased rapidly. A little later she reached another orgasm.

With difficulty she managed not to moan loudly, as she was used to. It took a long time for her to calm down again.

"Cedylein, you have something. I should be careful or I'll fall in love with you," she murmured.

She fell asleep with her hands between her legs.

Anna woke up first.

She still had one hand between her legs. She smiled as she thought about the previous night. It had been a good idea that she had crawled into his sleeping bag to warm up. Now she had to dispose of the condoms as quickly as possible before her brother woke up.

As quietly as possible she left the tent and went into the forest.

Yesterday's rain had brought about a strong cooling. The sun had not yet reached the valley floor. She found a place among the bushes and undid her pants.

In such moments she would like to be a man. Peeing standing up was definitely easier. After making sure she hadn't overlooked any nettles or prickly weeds, she crouched on the forest floor. She spread her thighs and emptied her full bladder. As she watched the beam, she thought back to last night.

Just the memory of sweet Cedric with the beautiful penis made her shudder. Waves of excitement raced over her body.

As beautiful as with Cedric, she had never experienced sexual intercourse.

The youngster had achieved something that none of her previous friends had achieved: an intense orgasm. So far she had always had to help out.

After she finished urinating, she pulled the knotted condoms out of her jacket pocket. She looked at the well-filled things with a smile. She hoped there would be a sequel.

With a small spoon she had brought with her, she digged a hole in the forest floor. She threw the condoms into the pit and closed it again with dirt.

Then she went back to the campsite and began clearing out her tent. She cursed loudly. Almost all of her clothes were wet. Just as she had hung everything up to dry, her mother came out of the tent sleepily.

"Good morning Anna."

"Good morning, mother. Slept well?"

"The little time that your father gave me, I slept well. And you? What are you doing there?"

"All my clothes got wet!"

"Will you help me with breakfast?"

"Sure, I'm coming."

After breakfast, Cedric helped with the dishes. Harry and his father examined the small, leaky tent.

Anna had gone to Mayrhofen to go shopping.

Harry's mother washed the dishes and then handed them to Cedric to dry.

"Do you like camping?"

"Yeah, it's even better than I thought."

"Do you miss your girlfriend? You have one?"

Cedric hesitated and felt himself blush.

"Uhh... no... I don't have a girlfriend."

"I don't understand, such a handsome and sweet boy."

Carolin sensed his embarrassment and changed the subject.

"I'm going to look for mushrooms later. Do you want to come along?"

"I don't know mushrooms. I would definitely only use poisonous ones."

"No problem! I'll show you what we're looking for."

"Then I'd like to come with you."

Harry and his father were still busy repairing Anna's tent.

"Will you be able to fix it?" Carolin asked her husband.

"I don't know, the seam ripped and we don't have real glue. I will talk to Anna, either she sleeps in our tent or we have to go to Munich and get a spare tent from the basement."

"Will it take you long?"

"I do not know why?"

"Cedric and I are going to look for mushrooms. Then I can prepare a delicious meal."

"That's a great idea. I love mushroom dishes."

She said goodbye to her husband with a tender kiss. Cedric followed her into the woods, basket in hand. Yesterday's storm had passed. The sun burned down from the sky; soon Cedric was bathed in sweat.

Carolin, on the other hand, didn't seem impressed.

After two hours they still hadn't found any mushrooms. Cedric was beginning to regret that he had gone with them. Carolin suggested taking a break. They sat on a fallen tree and took a breather.

"It is very hot today. You shouldn't believe that we had such a thunderstorm yesterday," she began a conversation.

Cedric looked past her into the valley.

"It was a heavy rain. Her husband explained to us that this is more common in the mountains."

"Yes, the weather changes very quickly."

Out of the corner of his eye, he watched his best friend's mother undo the top two buttons of her blouse. As she leaned forward, he could see deep into her cleavage.

She was clearly not wearing a bra!

Cedric felt himself blush with embarrassment.

Carolin pretended not to notice.

"We should move on. I always found mushrooms right up there. But before that I have to go into the bushes for a moment."

She got up and disappeared behind a small clump of bushes. Cedric looked after her, then he heard a soft splash. Shortly afterwards Martha returned.

She rubbed her bottom.

"It's easier for you men. I sat in a nettle. Let's go."

They continued up the mountain. As she had predicted, they soon found the first porcini mushrooms. Carolin showed him how to peel the valuable mushrooms out of the moss with a knife.

When he looked up, he had another great look at her blouse. He stopped cutting and secretly looked at her enormous bust size. Carolin noticed his eyes and grinned mischievously.

She hadn't unbuttoned her blouse for nothing!

"Do you like what you see?"

Cedric blushed. He swallowed and lowered his eyes.

"Yes," he stammered.

"I noticed the way you surreptitiously eyed me yesterday. You can do this openly. I like it when I please men."

The red spots on his cheeks grew even larger.

Carolin grinned at him.

"It's a compliment to an old woman like me when young men like my breasts. So, as long as we're alone here, you can look at my bust size unabashedly."

Carolin put the basket on its side and took the knife from his hand. Then she undid the last few buttons, took off her blouse and dropped it on the forest floor.

Her upper body was completely exposed!

Cedric looked stunned at the beautiful breasts. Her nipples were already stiff and sticking out at least an inch.

He had never seen such long nipples!

She took his hands and pulled him to a tree. She leaned against the trunk and put his hands on her breasts.

Cedric was stunned and didn't know what was happening to him.

"Are you satisfied now?"

He didn't know what to say.

Under his hands, the powerful nipples seemed to grow even more. He leaned over and kissed a nipple.

Carolin put her hands around his head and pressed him to her breasts.

"You can suck a little harder. I like that. It reminds me of when I breastfed my kids."

Slowly he followed her request and began to suck the big wart more and more. Suddenly she let go of his head.

Cedric feared that that would all be the end of it.

But when he looked up, he saw a mildly smiling face.

"You're doing fine. You're either natural or you had a good teacher."

Cedric stuttered.

"I... uh... don't have much experience."

Carolin smiled and leaned towards him. Softly but firmly, she placed her lips on his. Cedric flinched when he felt her tongue.

The tip of her tongue pushed gently through his lips. He gripped her plump breasts again and enjoyed the tongue game.

The kisses became more and more violent and demanding.

Cedric started when he felt her unzip his pants and pull them down. She gently grabbed his member and began stroking it.

He moaned as she grabbed his scrotum and squeezed hard.

"Let's swap places," she whispered. "Lean on the tree trunk."

He followed her instructions. As soon as he leaned against her, she got down on her knees and kissed his stiff penis. He watched in disbelief as his best friend's mom took his cock in her mouth.

He had only seen such things in porn movies before!

Soon he heard himself moaning loudly. He put his hand on her shoulders. Then he bent over her and tried to get to her breasts again. Astonished, he noticed that her nipples had grown even larger. He rubbed them between his fingers.

Startled, he let go of the nipples when Carolin moaned loudly.

"Excuse me, Ms. Plessen. I didn't mean to hurt them."

"You didn't hurt me. On the contrary, you do it very well."

He immediately cupped her hard nipple between his index finger and thumb. He squeezed, twisted and massaged her nipple considerably harder. He was so mesmerized by those beautiful breasts that he didn't realize how aroused he was already.

Suddenly he felt his climax approaching.

He let go of her breasts, leaned against the tree trunk and closed his eyes. Carolin worked his phallus more and more intensively and scratched his scrotum at the same time. This was better than he had imagined in his wildest dreams. Twice more she stopped and prevented his orgasm.

The third time, she increased her effort and massaged him so hard that he exploded, screaming loudly. He held her head and thrust deep into her mouth in quick succession. His sperm shot down her throat in violent spurts. She smiled at him and swallowed his seed. His knees were shaking and he was breathing heavily.

Caroline got up. Her tongue slid over her lips, removing the last traces of his warm load. She stroked her breasts with one hand. The other she had between her legs.

He slowly calmed down and came back to reality.

"That tasted good. Would you like to try it too?"

Cedric didn't know what she meant. He looked at her questioningly.

"I...uhh...don't quite understand..."

Carolin smiled as she stepped out of her skirt and then removed her panties.

"I have tried your sex, of course you have the same right if you want to."

He nodded hesitantly.

"That... uhh... I've never done that before. I don't know if I can."

"Thats is quite easy. Just try."

Cedric knelt in front of his best friend's naked mother. From a short distance he looked at her private parts. The first thing he saw was a dense triangle of black pubic hair.

The sight excited him. Slowly but steadily his body pumped blood into the erectile tissue of his cock.

Carolin watched the process; a smile played on her lips.

“You seem to like my hairy vagina. That makes a mature woman happy.”

She gave him a kiss, sat on the log and spread her legs.

For the first time in his life, Cedric was able to look between a woman's spread thighs. He liked what he saw better than in his porn films. He realized that her private hair was the same jet black color as the hair on her head.

"Come on, my young stallion. I want to feel your tongue."

Uncertain, Cedric approached the goal of his desire. Carolin squeezed and pulled on her long, stiff nipples.

"You can do anything you want. Just don't bite. I do not like it."

He looked at her in astonishment. "Why would I bite you?"

"Some men do that, but you can forget it in a moment."

As he leaned forward, a scent caught his nostrils, increasing his arousal even further. He gently stroked his fingertips through her pubic hair.

"You dare. You can't go wrong. If I don't like something, I'll tell you."

Cedric took a deep breath and let it out again. Watching porn movies was something completely different from reality. His curiosity awoke!

He pushed the dense hair aside and found her wet column.

The stimulating scent became more and more intense. He liked the smell and leaned forward to inhale more.

Carolin observed his still uncertain urge to explore with a smile. It felt exciting to see the young man examining her vulva.

The big surprise came when he pulled her pussy lips apart. A white, thin thread appeared!

Cedric looked up uncertainly.

"I thought you might enjoy removing my tampon. You just have to pull the string slowly."

He didn't need to be told twice!

Her sex slowly opened and the tampon became visible. Cedric didn't give up and soon had pulled him out completely. He briefly looked at the typically female utensil.

"Just drop him. And keep going. I like the way you touch me."

Cedric dropped the white part and fulfilled the dream of countless weighting fantasies. He stuck out his tongue and touched her labia. He had often wondered what that would taste like.

It was delicious!

Faster and faster he let his tongue slide over her crack.

"Uh, you're doing well," she moaned.

So encouraged, he dared more. His tongue slid faster and faster over her pussy lips while he pulled them further apart.

Her moans continued to fuel him.

He rubbed her wet vagina faster and harder.

She pressed his head tightly against her pleasure center. Cedric licked and sucked like his life was at stake. He would have preferred to never stop. Suddenly her legs broke away from him.

"Let me down. I want to feel you."

Carolin climbed down from the tree and took a large bath towel out of her backpack. Spreading it out, she lay on her back and spread her thighs.

"Come on. I want to feel you inside of me."

Cedric hurried to get between her legs. In contrast to the previous night, he scored on the first try and slid into the warm, damp crevice. Her muscles began an exciting dance around his member.

Since it hadn't been long since his last orgasms, he had more stamina. Her hands rested on his buttocks and rhythmically pressed him against her.

Cedric wavered between happiness and panic. He was afraid to come early again. As an experienced woman, Carolin sensed this immediately.

"If you're coming, just come. You don't need to hold back."

That was like a cue for him and he let himself fall into his orgasm. A few violent pelvic thrusts and he pumped his hot cum into her vagina.

Panting heavily, he dropped onto Carolin. He was just happy. She gently stroked his head.

"I liked that very much. You have a beautiful cock."

She turned to him and kissed his cheek.

Dark thoughts came over Cedric.

What if her husband found out?

Carolin seemed to have an inkling of the thoughts tormenting him.

"Now we have our little secret. I hope it's in good hands with you."

Cedric nodded. "I won't tell anyone."

She smiled at him. "We have to go back to the campsite now, otherwise the others will think we're lost."

She reached into her pocket, took out a tampon and held it out to him on her open hand

"Would you like to stick it in me?"

Cedric nodded. He hastily removed the cover. He pushed her labia apart and pushed the tampon deep into her vagina.

Caroline groaned.

"You are doing wonderfully. That leaves you wanting more."

On the way back he suddenly remembered that he had had sex with her without a condom. What if there were consequences.

He gathered all his courage.

"Mrs. Plessen, we didn't use rubber. What if there are consequences?"

She smiled at him.

"You should think about that next time. But no fear. I'm taking the pill."

She pulled him towards her and kissed him.

"You're a really sweet boy. How about we do a repeat tonight?"

Cedric stared at her in astonishment.

"How does that work? I'm sleeping in a tent with Harry. And what about her husband?"

Secretly he thought of Anna. What would his queen of hearts, his goddess, his secret love think?

"Let that be my concern. What is it, do you want to?"

Cedric nodded his head happily. "Oh yes, very much. You are a wonderful, very erotic woman."

"Okay, let's do one more round today."

She took his hand and only let him go when they were close to the campsite.

"Give me another kiss," she demanded.

They hugged and a kiss turned into a passionate, very erotic tongue game. By now he was losing his inhibitions. His hands kneaded her breasts.

Groaning, she broke away from him.

"Boy, you're one too. You're not going to be hard again are you?"

"Yes, I am," he announced proudly. And to add emphasis, he pressed his stiff member firmly against her body.

"Do you want to fuck me again quickly?"

Cedric swallowed and nodded his head.

She put the basket of mushrooms on the floor.

"Then show what you've got."

She turned, slowly pushed her skirt up provocatively, and leaned forward. He looked greedily at her plump ass. Carolin supported herself on a tree trunk and spread her legs.

He didn't want to miss this chance!

Fucking a woman standing from behind; another dream of his youth.

He freed his hard penis from the tightness of his pants. He happily grabbed the string and removed the tampon. Then he stood behind her, grabbed her pelvis and pushed his member between her legs.

Carolin moaned as he entered her deeply.

"Boy, boy, you have a mighty tribe."

He slowly began to push her. Her moans grew louder and louder. He leaned forward, reached under her blouse for her breasts and looked for the large nipples.

When he squeezed her nipple tightly and stretched it out, Carolin was overwhelmed by a violent orgasm.

Panting heavily, she reveled in the exhilaration that the boy gave her. She returned the favor with a vigorous massage of his member. Carolin knew the effects of her vaginal muscles.

She didn't have to wait long to get confirmation.

With a long drawn out 'Ahh' his sperm shot into her warm lust cavity.

Only slowly did the intoxication of the feelings subside.

"You're really insatiable. I think that's enough. We have to make sure we come back."

He was reluctant to break away from her. Both of them quickly put their clothes in order. She kissed him on the cheek.

"That was a nice ending to mushroom picking."

Soon after, they were back at the campsite. Her husband was already waiting for her.

"Did you find something?"

Carolin waved the full basket.

“We were successful. We found some great porcini mushrooms."

She hugged her husband like a newlywed couple.

After dinner, Harry's father explained that he wanted to go back to Munich that night. Anna's tent was so broken that it could not be repaired. He had a spare tent in the basement at home. Anna also wanted to ride as the flooding had soaked most of her clothes. She wanted to get spare clothes. Harry decided to go too; so he could spend a night with his girlfriend in Munich.

Cedric couldn't believe his luck!

He would be left alone at the campsite with Harry's mother!

After the meal, the three left and promised to be back the next day by lunchtime.

Carolin and Cedric took care of the dishes and got the tents in shape. Then they sat tired in front of the campfire.

Carolin had opened a bottle of wine and Cedric had a beer.

"Well, what do you say? Now we have the whole night to ourselves."

Cedric nodded enthusiastically.

"You could almost say they planned it."

"But I haven't. I wouldn't have managed it that perfectly," she answered with a grin.

Cedric got up and sat down behind her and wrapped his arms around her body. Carolin put her glass aside and leaned her head back.

Then she noticed that she was getting cold. The sun had long since set, the stars shone in the night sky.

Cedric started kissing her neck and placed his hands on her thighs. Carolin enjoyed his tenderness. When he placed his hands on her breasts, she shuddered.

It was now completely dark. Cedric stopped his stroking.

"I have to go."

Carolin nodded into the darkness. "I also. Let's go pee."

She pulled him behind her to the nearby edge of the forest.

"Come on," she asked him with a grin.

"But that's not possible," he answered nervously.

"Should I help you?"

"Uhh... I don't understand..." he stammered.

"Turn around," she instructed.

Cedric turned his back on her and looked into the forest. Carolin stepped behind him, embraced his body and opened his trousers. She gently pulled down his jeans and pulled his penis out of his panties.

She pulled back his foreskin and aimed it at a tree.

"Let's see a nice bow."

It took Cedric a while before he complied with her wish. He closed his eyes and focused on the pressure in his bladder. Then he felt his urine spurting out of his penis.

He leaned against Carolin and enjoyed this intimate moment. When she had shaken off the last drops, she pushed his penis back into her panties.

Then she took a step back, reached under her skirt and pulled off her panties.

With a grin, she lowered herself and spread her thighs.

"Do you have to pee too, Mrs. Plessen?" he asked.

"Sure, I have to."

"May I watch them? Help them? "

"Whatever you want."

Cedric walked around her and knelt behind the woman. He grabbed her slender body, pulled up her skirt and stroked her thick pubic hair. He gently squeezed the area where he suspected her blister.

Carolin gasped softly and surrendered to her urge. As soon as the first drops fell on the floor, she felt his hand pressed firmly against her labia.

Cedric was amazed by the warm stream that washed over his hand. He massaged her harder and harder. Even when her bladder was completely empty. Carolin began to moan in pleasure as he shoved a finger into her wet slit. He increased the pressure, began penetrating her faster.

Carolin supported herself on the floor and lifted her pelvis.

His finger movements became faster and faster.

Then he felt her body tremble.

She cried out in pleasure as the orgasm rolled over her body.

It took a while for her body to calm down. She had never had so much eroticism and satisfaction in one day.

She got up and straightened her clothes.

"Come on, let's go back to the tent," she said, taking his hand. "We don't want to catch a cold."

A little later they sat in front of the campfire and warmed up. Carolin drained the bottle of wine while they talked animatedly.

"I'm going to sleep now, Cedric," she explained, but her voice sounded slightly slurred. "Good night."

She got up and went into the big main tent.

Cedric looked after her in amazement because he had hoped for nocturnal sex. But Harry's mother seemed drunk and tired.

However, he wasn't tired yet. This day had been the most exciting in his life so far. He got himself another bottle of beer, sat in front of the campfire and enjoyed the starry sky.

From the main tent he heard loud snoring. Carolin seemed sound asleep. That made him curious.

He quietly crept into her tent.

She was wrapped in a dark blue sheepsack and appeared to be sound asleep. He looked around Harry's parents' bedroom.

Suddenly saw a black vibrator and a skin-colored dildo lying on the edge. So far he had only seen something like this on the Internet. Curiously, he examined the two toys. Especially the vibrator aroused his interest.

Again and again he looked at the sleeping Carolin, but she hadn't noticed his presence. She snored like a Russian wandering puff.

He quietly crept to her sleeping bag and unzipped it. When this was open, he could unfold the fabric completely. Carolin slept completely naked!

He gently spread her legs and could see that her labia opened slightly with this movement.

That awakened his curiosity!

He got the vibrator and spread lube on the toy.

With one hand he pushed her labia apart and pressed the artificial pleasure dispenser against her column. He slowly pushed the sex toy into her wet grotto. Then he grabbed the remote control and turned on the vibrator. Little by little he tried out all the functions.

"What are you doing there?"

Cedric was startled.

He hadn't noticed that Carolin had woken up and was watching him with curious eyes.

"I... uhh... excuse me, Ms. Plessen," he stammered.

"You're doing fine. Where did you get the practice?"

"I do not have any. It's the first vibrator I've ever seen."

"Keep going."

Carolin closed her eyes and began to massage her breasts. She was sure that Cedric didn't need any help.

He continued to play with the remote control and did it so skillfully that Carolin was soon moaning loudly. He slowly increased the intensity of the vibrator.

Shortly thereafter she reached her climax.

Her body trembled, her pulse raced, her eyes went black, the feelings were so intense.

When she opened her eyes again, the vibrator was gone. Cedric knelt naked between her spread thighs and stroked his hard cock.

"Fuck me please," she breathed excitedly.

He leaned forward, pushed his penis between her parted labia and gently penetrated her. Carolin wrapped her legs around his back and pressed her body against his erection.

They quickly found the same rhythm.

In and out, in and out.

Always deeper, harder and more intense.

A little later Cedric reached his peak.

He pumped his warm sperm into her vagina again and again, thrust after thrust. When she felt this, she got the second climax within a few minutes.

Around noon the next day, the three returned from Munich. Harry and his father cleared out the car and shortly thereafter began to set up the small replacement tent.

Cedric helped Anna with her luggage.

"Cedy, we need to talk," she whispered softly in his ear. He looked at her in amazement.

"What do we need to discuss?"

Anna put her hand on his.

"Would you like to go for a little hike in the mountains? We could have a great chat."

"Yes, of course," he beamed. "I am very pleased."

Two hours later they were already on the Hollenzberg and had a wonderful view over the Zillertal. Directly below them was Mayrhofen, to their right Zell am Ziller, to their left Finkenberg with the mighty Tux Glacier.

At an altitude of almost 1,600 meters it was pleasant, the sun wasn't burning as hard as in the valley.

Anna had spread out a blanket in a meadow to the side of the hiking trail. She took a bottle of water out of her backpack and handed it to Cedric.

"Why are you looking at me so thoughtfully?" he asked curiously.

"It must be the butterflies in my stomach."

Cedric looked at her questioningly.

"I do not understand what you mean."

"I did a lot of thinking on the long drive. Cedric, I fell in love with you."

She gave him a kiss on the cheek.

Cedric couldn't believe that such a pretty girl fell in love with him. Her gaze made his pulse race too.

"Do you really mean that?"

"Of course, Cedylein," she replied gently. "It's no fun with something like that. What do you say?"

"I fell in love with you too," he replied. "It was five years ago in September."

"I beg your pardon?"

"In September five years ago I was at your house with Harry for the first time. You were sixteen then and the most beautiful girl in the world. When I first saw you, I fell in love with you. It only took about ten seconds! I've only dreamed of you for five years. I've never had a girlfriend as I've compared every girl to you but none could compete with you."

"You've loved me for five years?"

"Yes," he said embarrassed, looking at the floor. Between his fingers he played with the lush grass of the Alpine slopes.

"You are sweet."

Anna laid her head on his chest. She enjoyed the tingling of his fingers stroking her long hair.

Again she compared him to her previous friends. She came to the same conclusion again: Cedric was completely different, he was clearly very special. She felt completely happy.

"Anna?"

"Yes, cedyle?"

"I do not know how to say it. Do you mind that I'm younger?"

"No, why should it bother me?"

"What will your friends say?"

"I'm sure they'll tease me a little, but I don't care. They don't know what I have in you. And believe me, if they make fun of you, then they can experience something. Don't worry, they won't eat you. You'll get to know her soon, by the way. My best friend is having a big garden party in three weeks. It's always a big party."

She put a hand on his stomach and slowly moved it to his pants. Tenderly she stroked the fabric and felt his erection.

Cedric could have stayed like that for hours, but the weather gods had no understanding. A cloud moved in front of the sun and shortly afterwards it started to rain.

They quickly packed up and fled into the valley. Hand in hand they stumbled down the slope. Cedric noticed an overhanging rock and pulled Anna towards it. As soon as they reached the dry place, the rain became even heavier. They sat down on a stone that leaned against the rock face like a bench and wrapped themselves in the warm blanket.

Tenderly she stroked her black hair from her forehead.

"It's a nice place, if only I wasn't so cold."

Cedric looked at her in surprise. "I'm not cold."

He put his arm around her shoulders and hugged her tightly. They watched the rain, which was getting heavier and heavier, tightly embraced.

A loud thunder made both jump. Flash after flash followed faster and faster. The storm seemed to have caught up in the Zillertal.

Cedric watched the spectacle while Anna snuggled closer and closer to him. His hand ran incessantly down her back, sometimes down her neck as well.

Anna put her hand on his thigh and started stroking his jeans. She placed her hand on his erection and massaged the bulge.

"Would you please take off your pants?" she asked in a whisper. "Then I can caress you better," she continued when she noticed his puzzled look.

“Gladly, but equal rights for both. I would be happy if you take off your jeans too.”

With warm feelings in her stomach, Anna thought that none of her friends had ever asked her anything so kindly. They would have simply unzipped her pants and stripped off the fabric.

"You're cute," she breathed.

Both got up and opened their trousers. Almost in the same rhythm they stripped off their clothes.

"The rest too, Cedylein. Please!"

He smiled at her, grabbed his panties and pulled them down. She watched his every move and admired the masculine form of his sex. His penis looked even more attractive than she had imagined. In the darkness of last night she had only been able to feel him but not see him.

"I like what I see," she breathed, smiling softly.

"Now you! Please, I want to see your body."

"You lecher," she answered with a grin and kissed him lovingly on the mouth.

Then she took a step back so that he could see her well.

Se undid the buttons of her blouse and stripped them off. Then she took off her bra.

Cedric took a deep breath and exhaled as he took in the perfect shape of her bust. In her beauty, Anna seemed to him like a goddess who had just left Olympus.

She was perfect!

With a teasing grin on her lips, she grabbed the waistband of her panties and slowly pulled them down. When the panties reached the floor, she strode towards Cedric.

"Sit down, please," she asked him.

He laid the blanket on the stone and sat down. Anna crawled over his thighs and snuggled into his lap.

His penis was already sticking out hard from his body in its full size without any external influence. Anna edged closer and closer to him. When their lips found a passionate kiss, his stiff member touched her slightly parted labia.

"I love you, Cedy," she moaned, ramming his penis deep into her privates in one firm motion.

Cedric enjoyed the friction in her vagina, but he enjoyed the eye contact even more. He thought he was penetrating through her pupils into her soul and touching her true "I".

Anna moved faster and faster, but maintained eye contact. She saw his eyes turn from a shade of brown to a dark green.

Only when her moans got louder and she started to move wildly did she break eye contact. Anna thought she was flying through the universe, past the shining stars, the orgasm flowed through her body so intensely

Her climax started at her big toe, raced through her legs, up her torso, and exploded in her brain. She trembled, wailed, moaned and lost touch with her surroundings.

As she opened the door to the present again, she felt his warm cum dripping out of her vagina. During her journey through the universe he had poured himself into her.

"Cedy, that was great."

"I love you, Anna," he breathed, kissing her cheek and nibbling on her left earlobe.

"I love you too, honey," she replied. "We should remember this position, I've never felt an orgasm so intensely."

As soon as they were fully dressed, a hunting dog ran up and shortly afterwards a hunter under a thick rain jacket.

"Hello, are you lost?"

"No, let's wait under that ledge until the rain stops. We live at the Mayrhofen campsite."

"Wait for the rain? But you will have to wait a long time. The rain will hardly stop today.

The hound sat down next to Cedric and leaned on his legs. Even when his master called him, he looked up briefly, but just sat there.

The hunter acknowledged his dog's behavior with a smile.

"I guess you like dogs. Otherwise it wouldn't stick to you like that."

Cedric shook his head: "Actually, I'm more afraid of strange dogs."

"You should hurry and run to the valley. We are having a calmer rainy season right now, but the thunderstorm will intensify."

"Thank you," Anna replied, taking Cedric's hand. Together they hurried down the trail into the valley.

They arrived at the campsite completely soaked.

They spent the afternoon in the main tent playing various card games.

Since grilling was out of the question, they drove to Finkenberg for dinner. In the tavern that evening there was a party from the local costume association, which made Harry snort contemptuously. The thought of having to listen to folk music all evening made him gloomy.

Therefore, after dinner, he urged an immediate departure.

By the time they reached Mayrhofen, the rain had almost stopped. So they could have a drink together under the awning.

Cedric had no idea that two women would have liked to spend the night with him. After an hour of pleasant conversation, each of the men had already downed three bottles of beer.

Cedric knocked out the fourth bottle Harry wanted to hand him.

"No thanks, I'm already tired. I'll quickly go out into the forest again and then sleep in our tent."

After a few steps he heard someone following him.

He turned and recognized Anna. She took his hand and quickly pulled him on.

"We do not have much time. Harry will be right there."

After a few steps she stopped and hugged him. They quickly began kissing. Cedric put his hands around her waist and hugged her tightly.

A cracking branch threw them apart. Her father passed a few meters from them without noticing her. Just behind him followed a slightly swaying Harry.

They slipped quietly to the side. Behind a thick tree they hoped to remain unnoticed. But there was no time for more than a few kisses.

When Cedric came into the tent, Harry was already in his sleeping bag and had immersed himself in one of his porn magazines.

"You have to see those monster tits!"

Cedric internally moaned!

That's exactly what he had feared. Harry would now go through the whole booklet with him. All he wanted was to lie down in his sleeping bag and dream of Anna.

But Harry had no understanding, slid closer and showed him the pictures.

Suddenly someone knocked on the tarpaulin.

"It's me, Anna. May I come in? The new tent is also leaking. It's raining on me."

"Of course," Harry replied, quickly hiding the porn magazines.

Anna crawled into the tent with her sleeping bag.

"Thanks, that's nice of you. I don't feel like sleeping in the main tent. Mom snores so loudly."

She threw the sleeping bag between Cedric and the tent wall. She carefully crawled into the tent and crawled into the warm cavity of her sleeping bag.

Harry turned off the flashlight and turned to face away.

Anna stretched out her hand to Cedric and gently stroked his face. He kissed her fingertips and wished Harry would fall asleep quickly. But that didn't seem to be the case today, he kept tossing and turning. Suddenly he grunted and peeled himself out of his sleeping bag. Anna waited until he had left the tent.

"Yes, yes, the beer."

Cedric nodded. "I haven't seen him that drunk in a long time."

"It's a pity that my tent is so small. Otherwise you could have come to me."

"I thought your tent was leaking?"

"It was a white lie. Otherwise I would have to sleep alone. You wouldn't have come to me, would you? "

Cedric bit her finger.

"You are one to me. But it's not true. I wanted to come as soon as Harry was asleep."

"He'll be asleep soon, drunk as he is. I'll tell you one thing, if you drink that much, then it's over with us."

"I have no problem with that, I don't like alcohol.

"That's good because I've had bad experiences with drunk men."

The return of Harry ended their conversation. After he turned off the flashlight again, Anna pulled Cedric's hand towards her and returned the tenderness she had previously received.

Harry had no idea what was going on that was happening so close to him. He thought they were both sound asleep and decided to leaf through a porn magazine by flashlight. In order not to wake up the others, he crept deep into the sleeping bag and thus covered the light.

Unlike Cedric, Anna had no idea what kind of literature kept her brother awake. But soon she knew what he was doing, because even his muffled moans could not be ignored.

Anna found the situation funny but also exciting at the same time.

Suddenly it was quiet in the tent. The weak glow of the flashlight went out and shortly afterwards a soft snoring showed that Harry had finally started his way to dreamland.

They lay still for a while. Then Anna couldn't stand it in her sleeping bag anymore. Cedric was already waiting for her.

As they kissed, they began to undress each other. There was no trace of his shyness the last time. They pushed each other down their pants with their feet. It didn't all happen without laughter.

Suddenly Harry wheezed.

"Can't you be quiet. I want to sleep."

"Me too, just remembered a joke from earlier."

"Joker," Harry growled and fell asleep again in a moment.

Anna pressed her slim, soft body greedily against Cedric. She kissed slowly from the neck down his chest and down. Finally she had reached her goal!

Softly she breathed a kiss on the steeply rising limb.

Cedric groaned softly.

She wrapped her lips around his penis and smackingly began to suck his head while she put one hand between her thighs and intensely massaged her clit.

She gently scraped his skin with her fingernails until she reached his scrotum. She tickled the swollen balls with her fingertips. Then she took a testicle between three fingers and moved it back and forth.

Her tongue caressed the underside of his bare glans. With her teeth she nibbled tenderly at the head of his shaft.

Cedric reared up with pleasure, whereupon Anna let her tongue circle around his glans even faster. He drew a deep, loud breath into his lungs as she took the tip of his cock between her lips.

His member slowly entered her mouth. Cedric kept trying to jerk his pelvis forward in order to get in deeper. But

Anna was able to dodge it skillfully. Her tongue twirled on his underside, seeking the tender spots. Further and further she pushed his hard piece into her mouth until she had absorbed him completely. She felt his glans on the roof of her mouth and began to suck lightly. One hand tickled his balls, the other hand scraped the sharp fingernails up towards his stomach. You feel his tense abdominal muscles.

A twitch went through his body.

She had reached her goal and felt his approaching orgasm. Even faster she sucked on his wand. She wanted him to erupt in her mouth.

The helpless Cedric exploded and pumped all his cum down her throat. She swallowed it all and savored the pleasant taste of his semen.

After licking his cock clean, she crawled up into his arms. She snuggled tiredly into his shoulder.

"If Harry knew what we were doing, he'd be sober in no time," she whispered.

"He would surely watch."

“Yes, my brother is a born voyeur. He keeps trying to watch me shower. But I've never let him see more than my butt. I was hoping that that would happen once he had a steady girlfriend. But nothing has changed.”

"If I had such a beautiful sister, I would try too."

"I'm glad you're not my brother."

"I also."

Anna gave him a gentle kiss.

"Goodnight My Dear. Sleep well."

Cedric was too excited to sleep. He stroked Anna until she was sound asleep.

Harry groaned the next morning.

"Oh god, I feel sick."

Cedric rubbed his eyes sleepily. "Just drink less."

Harry's response was unprintable. He fled the tent without closing it behind him.

The damp cold crept in through the opening. Cedric considered staying in bed, but hunger made him crawl out of his sleeping bag. He dressed quickly and hurried through the rain to the main tent.

A good breakfast would make the day look rosier.

"Good morning, Cedric. Sit down. The tea will be ready soon."

Carolin winked at him with a smile and turned to the gas cooker. Cedric sat down next to Harry's father and began spreading Nutella on a roll.

Shortly thereafter, Marcel Plessen got up, grabbed his cigarettes and left the main tent.

"I'm outside for a smoke," he said goodbye.

"We heard you last night," Carolin said when her husband was gone.

"Did I snore?"

"No, Harry did the part."

Cedric needed a few seconds before he understood what Carolin meant for noises. He felt his cheeks flush with a flush of red. Now he was the shy boy again.

"Is okay. It's nice when you're young and in love. Did you have sex with my daughter?"

"Uhh... no not really," he replied, embarrassed.

"Ah, I see," she replied, nodding her head. "She gave you head to put you to sleep. Men like that, I know that from Marcel."

"Yeah... uhh."

Somehow Cedric felt embarrassed talking to Anna's mother about her daughter's oral activities.

"You've blushed, Cedric," she said, grinning. "I don't even know you like that. Can you please wake up Anna?"

"Yes, of course, Mrs. Plessen."

Cedric, still red in the face, turned and hurriedly left the tent. Marcel stood in front of the tent and drew on his cigarette.

"Next time you'll get your own, slightly larger tent. Then you'll be more comfortable."

He quickly ran through the rain to his tent. Anna slept deeply and soundly. She didn't notice that he crawled into the tent. Her long, blue-black hair framed her head like a halo.

He lay down next to her and kissed her cheek.

"What time is it?"

"Nearly ten o'clock. you overslept I'm supposed to wake you up, breakfast is already ready."

She opened her sleeping bag and dressed quickly. Holding hands, they went to their parents' tent. Harry was still so busy with his nausea that he didn't notice.

Completely different from his parents.

Marcel nodded to the two and pushed them the bread that had just been spread.

"Good morning Anna. Unfortunately, it looks like we're going to go home after all.

I just heard the weather forecast. It's supposed to rain continuously for the next few days. That's not how camping is fun. Is everyone okay if we go home?"

They unanimously agreed to his proposal.

Harry skipped breakfast. He kept oscillating between tent and forest. The color of his face improved only slowly.

After breakfast they began to dismantle the tents. Carolin and Cedric met when giving away.

On the drive home, Anna sat back in the middle and held Cedric's hand.

About three hours later they reached Munich.

Would their love endure despite the age difference?

2

BET WON!

Finally I stood in front of the apartment door and desperately looked for the key. I cursed inwardly and made a mental note to finally tidy my purse like I had a hundred thousand times before. Of course it would remain a pious wish this time too.

After some searching and fiddling, the time had come and I stood in the hallway of my parents' house. We lived in a terraced house in the Pasing district of Munich.

It was the end of July and I was on semester break. I studied art history and musicology at the University of Innsbruck. I had specifically decided to go to Austria because I had to experience an unpleasant separation after my Abitur. So the physical distance to Munich was good for me.

I dragged the trolley case behind me to my room and flopped down on the bed. It was so quiet in this house, very different from the dormitory where I stayed.

Shortly thereafter I opened my suitcase, took out the toiletry bag and the dirty laundry and went into the bathroom. The used clothes disappeared into the laundry bucket and immediately afterwards I threw my t-shirt, my socks and my panties.

I stood completely naked in the green tiled room and thought, as so often, that the architect should be strangled for his color choice.

I took a quick look at myself in the mirror and realized I looked tired.

Just freshen up!

After the shower, I went naked to my room and slipped under the covers. My mother had freshly made my bed.

I closed my eyes as if by myself and began to stroke my nipples tenderly with my right hand. I was tired, but I also knew

I wouldn't be able to sleep without relieving myself first.

I got up with a sigh and took my little black vibrator out of my closet. I checked its function before slipping back into my bed. I laid the blanket next to me as I liked being able to watch myself masturbate. I love the sight of the vibrator penetrating my vagina.

I spread my thighs greedily, caressing my blond pubic hair with my love servant. Then I slowly pushed it into my wet column.

He slipped easily into me, as if he had already been expected. I slowly fucked myself with the dildo. Immediately my nipples stiffened and grew into little towers. With my left hand I kneaded my breasts, with my right hand I guided the humming helper deep into my dripping vagina.

No, I literally rammed it in my cunt!

With maximum performance!

So I climbed the ladder of lust.

I was no longer aware of anything outside my room. A mistake, as it soon turned out!

Groaning, I enjoyed the humming tip on my clitoris. I screamed, gasped and tossed and turned.

My orgasm slowly subsided.

When I opened my eyes, I saw a dark shadow in the hallway. I widened my eyes in surprise!

Caught!

There stood Henri, my brother's twenty-year-old friend. I've known him for over five years. He was in and out of our house and spent all his free time with my brother Lukas.

Startled, I closed my legs, but I had forgotten the vibrator, which made itself felt and forced me to open my thighs again.

The little devil in me, however, immediately took over and I did something that I would not otherwise have thought of in life.

Spreading my thighs as wide as I could, I slowly pulled the vibrator out of my vagina and brought it to my mouth, where I began to lick it. My mucus was sweet and smelled intensely of orgasm.

I left my thighs open so Henri had a good view of my labia, which were slowly closing again.

He stood there, glued to his feet, watching me. I saw the bulge growing in his pants.

Only when my orgasm had subsided and the vibrator had been licked clean did I close my legs and sit up.

His eyes left my abdomen and focused on my face.

"Er..." he started to stammer. "Sorry... I didn't mean to..."

"But you did!" I replied pointedly and reproachfully.

“I... wanted... just... uhhh. I saw someone in the house and I thought it was your brother."

"Have you noticed that there is a bell on our house?"

"Yes...uh...I know that, but the front door was open."

Damn!

I forgot to close the door behind me.

He still didn't take his eyes off me. He literally took in the sight of my body. My slender, bent legs, my young, firm tits and stiff nipples.

The devil still had possession of me.

"Do you like what you see?"

"Uh..."

In slow motion, he turned his head away and mumbled, "'sorry."

He was about to leave when I called him back.

"Stop! Henri, come back at once!"

My request came in a sharp voice. He crept back to my door and looked at me like a miserable mess. He looked down in embarrassment, like a student caught smoking in the school bathroom.

"What else is it?" he mumbled.

"Come here. Now!" I ordered very dominantly.

His concerned and puzzled expression gave way to surprise. He probably wouldn't have expected such a tone.

"You want me to... come inside...?"

"Yes!"

He trotted in and stopped about a meter in front of me.

"Come a little closer!"

He came within arm's length and tried, with limited success, to cover up his curiosity. His eyes slid greedily over my body.

"You haven't answered my question yet!"

"What..." he swallowed. "What question...?"

Poor Henri was so caught off guard he really couldn't remember what I had asked him.

"I asked you if you liked what you see."

Now Henri took the time to examine my body in detail. Apparently he took that as permission to gawk at me.

"Uhh... yes... of course! You are beautiful, Naomi."

I reached out with my left arm and pressed her against the bulge in his pants from below.

"Not more?"

What was the matter with me?

Like a cat happily chasing a mouse, I took it upon myself and didn't give it a chance to escape.

"Yes... of course..."

"Of course what?"

I increased the pressure on his pants, causing his cock to continue to grow.

"You're very... sexy... a real blonde, I didn't know that," he explained after looking at my blonde pubic hair.

"Do you like pubic hair?"

"Oh yes, very much. Completely naked looks like a small child. But I'm not a pedophile."

"Are you so aroused by my pubic hair?"

"Not only that, your entire body is sexy."

I slammed my hand on the bulge, which he acknowledged with a cry of pain.

"So that gives you the right to gape at me and get horny, you horny pig?"

I increased the pressure on his hard cock.

"No, of course not," he immediately admitted sheepishly.

"Okay," I replied after a moment's thought. "I think we can make a little deal. After you've watched me do it to myself, it's only fair that I get to watch you do it like you do masturbate right?"

"You want me to jerk off here in front of you...uhhh...masturbate?" he came out in disbelief.

"That or I'll tell my mother that you lecher sneaked into our house to watch me secretly. Then you will be banned from here!"

"No, please don't," he replied anxiously.

"Then you'd better do as I say," I said sharply.

Still rather reluctantly he followed my instructions. His hands went to the belt and undid it. I took my hand off the bulge and waited for him to pull off his pants.

When I saw the tent in his panties, I couldn't help but lick my dry lips with my tongue.

Damn, I realized I was horny!

My orgasm from just now hadn't really contributed to the relief, but only made me even hornier. At my place of study I would have gone a few rooms further on such an occasion and would have had a good fuck with one of my friends.

Only my brother's friend was available to me here!

As he slipped off his panties, his stiff cock shot out and bobbed in my direction. His penis was aimed dangerously at my face.

Involuntarily I parted my thighs and stroked my blond pubic hair with the fingers of my left hand. The right hand played with my tits.

"Will I make you horny if I do this?"

"You make me horny since I first saw you five years ago," he replied.

What did he mean by that?

Shit, has my brother's friend been horny with me for so long?

He stared at me with wide eyes. His gaze swept between my breasts and crotch as his right hand closed around his cock, jerking it off frantically.

I saw his desperate efforts to a quick climax to get away from me.

"Stop!"

My voice echoed loudly across the room. My brother's friend stared at me in shock.

"That will not do! You move so fast I don't even notice!"

Obediently, Henri now tried to jerk off a little more slowly. The red acorn fascinated me. Whenever she emerged from the foreskin, the small slit opened. Thick veins ran through the love pole under the tip of his penis. In the wrinkled scrotum, the two balls bounced up and down with every movement.

I couldn't watch this any longer.

The moisture shot up in my vagina and was already dripping onto the bed.

I put my left hand on his right hand and slowly pulled it away from his cock. His phallus twitched towards me. I took his scrotum in my hand and massaged it tenderly.

"Ohhh... ahhh! Naomi, what are you doing?" he groaned, then stopped whimpering as I gripped his balls a little tighter.

"I'll do what I want!" I hissed.

Then I took the swollen tip of his penis in my mouth. I greedily suckled on this forbidden fruit and savored the salty-tart taste. I took my right hand out of my lap and wrapped it around the shaft of his bolt.

His breathing grew louder, more rattling.

I watched his reactions closely. The list of guys I'd screwed was long enough to realize that he was about to be there. Now the question arose how to proceed.

I was horny, that was for sure!

The only fuckable guy around was standing in front of me with his pants down and his cock in my mouth.

would i regret it

I had to buy time.

So I let go of his rod, leaned back and spread my legs.

"Now return the favor and lick my pussy!"

It was mean to starve him so close to his climax, but I needed time to think.

It was my brother's best friend!

A young boy of eighteen whom I had known for years.

Better if I ended this right now.

But I had to acknowledge that Henri has taken care of me well so far. His tongue was nimble and quick.

Damned!

He could lick really well!

Did he fuck as well as he licked?

There was only one way to find out!

"Mmmmm! You're doing well," I praised the young man.

In fact, he lifted his head and smiled lovingly and tenderly at me.

Was he in love with me?

Shit, I really should stop here or I'd break his heart too. That would definitely be bad for my karma!

But he had already pushed his tongue back into my crack.

Damn! I could also cleanse my karma in my next life.

"Do you want to fuck me?"

My brother's best friend hesitated only briefly.

"Yeah, yeah...uhh."

"But?"

"Are you sure you want this? You haven't even noticed me for the last few years and now you want sex with me?"

"The problem with you men is, you talk too much!"

Henri got up slowly.

His thick, stiff cock bobbed up and down in front of him. He looked delicious! The glans pointed exactly to my half-opened vagina out of sheer anticipation.

"Come!"

It was just one word. I took my labia in both hands and pulled them apart.

"She is waiting for you! Come fuck me!"

Henri was only a man, which means his blood had gone to his abdomen. As a result, there was an undersupply in his brain. I could have asked anything of him!

In no time he was completely undressed. He was very well built, lean, muscular, an eighteen-year-old Adonis.

Delicious!

He crawled onto my bed and lay between my legs. I took his hard cock and guided it to my blond haired cunt. With a single push he rammed his cock into my pleasure cave.

I leaned back and closed my eyes.

Then something happened that I didn't expect.

Most of the guys had started fucking me hard, banging me like a lovestruck rabbit.

Not so Henry!

My brother's eighteen-year-old friend was in control.

He took it slow, rotating his pelvis, thrusting his cock into every corner of my vagina.

Heaven! Was that good!

"Mhmmmm..." I growled, "...yeah...fine! Go on!"

His left hand grabbed my right breast, flexing it, playing with it, caressing it, twirling the nipple, without even stopping his horny thrusts.

A multifunctional fucker! Cool!

Our faces drew closer and our lips touched. I opened my mouth and let out my tongue. He sucked on it greedily. The warmth of lust flooded my body.

"Henry! Henry! I didn't think you could do that!"

Kissing we fucked each other more impetuously. In my opinion, he should actually be about to leave. But I wasn't ready yet!

Noticing it, he wrapped his arms around me and rolled us both around so I was lying on top of him. I gratefully took the opportunity to ride on his mighty pole. So I gave him the chance to grab my tits, take turns putting them in his mouth and caressing them.

My ride became ever sharper, my excitement grew ever greater.

Now it was me who was about to climax.

I knew what I wanted.

So I laid on top of him and turned us back into the missionary position. Henri saw what I wanted.

He began to fuck me calmly and deeply, always making sure his cock touched my sensitive areas near the clitoris.

"Mhmmm," I growled again. "Fuck me harder!"

As requested, he increased the pace. His thick cock plowed through my cunt like a steam hammer. I couldn't believe the stamina he had! He fucked me deep and hard and my lust increased at the same speed.

I was only moments away from my climax when he raised his pelvis and changed the angle at which he thrust into me.

I sucked in a sharp breath as his cock hit my g-spot.

"Ohhh... yeahaaaa!"

I wasn't able to do more, because now all that followed was my gasping. My desire increased with every thrust and it only took a short time until the waves finally crashed over me. Like a buck he hammered his cock into me and I was only too happy to give myself to him.

I climaxed, whimpering, until he suddenly sat up and motioned for me to turn around.

I was still not in control of my senses and complied with his request awkwardly.

As soon as I offered him my rear end, he put his cock on my vagina and pushed it in as deep as possible. He fucked me from behind. I felt like a bitch in heat. This position allowed his wonderful penis to penetrate areas of my body that had never been touched by a man before.

I can no longer say how long he used me. I missed those seconds because I was still enjoying my fading orgasm.

Suddenly he started to twitch and pumped his sperm into my pussy. The pleasant warmth of his love juice spread in my stomach. After a few more pushes, it was all over for him. He rolled onto his side and pulled me with him until we were lying next to each other in the spooning position.

Our breathing was difficult

Suddenly I heard noises in the hallway!

My younger brother Lukas stood in the doorway and grinned at us.

"Everything went really well, Henri. By the way, you looked hot when you were shagging."

"What?" I asked completely confused. I was speechless.

"The betting odds were so high that he couldn't refuse. For two years, the bets have been on when Henri will be able to fuck you. I took amazing pictures with my iPhone as proof. You haven't noticed how long I've been watching you."

"No... it can't... not..." I stammered.

"Hurry up Henri. We should take care of the betting winnings."

Henri got up and dressed.

Before he left my room, he kissed me softly on the cheek again.

"You're cute, Naomi. I would have fucked you without a bet."

Then I realized that I hadn't forgotten to close the front door. The two boys had already been waiting for me.

It had been a set up game to win a bet!

3

WOODED GORGES IN SWITZERLAND!

Every year, when it's slowly getting warmer again, I look forward to the summer camp in Switzerland. The past few years have always been very nice weeks. The first time I was still a teenager myself, this is where I had my first sexual experiences and I still feel very comfortable here in the great outdoors.

But the tide has turned!

Now I'm allowed to hang around with the adolescents during the day and make sure they don't do what I did back then. I still know them all, these tricks and secret hiding places. My target group is also different now: the carers.

It impresses women tremendously when you can deal with children. That's half the battle for a quickie.

If you also look charming and fit, nothing can really go wrong.

I was most keen on Lisa!

She is the younger sister of my best friend Tobias. Like every year, she organized this trip for the local church. Since we grew up almost like siblings due to my friendship with Tobias, I knew her physical development. She went from being a plain, flat-chested girl to a very erotic and beautiful young woman.

When I reached the meeting point, Lisa was already there. She was always very conscientious about the organization.

From a safe distance, I eyed her as she stood there on the bus with her list of participants. Her sweet angelic face and especially her small but prominent breasts, which were visible under the shirt, immediately cast a spell over me. It was quite a small breast, but it suited her and was shown to its best advantage by her delicate physique. She had tied her long blonde hair in a ponytail. She has a fantastic figure, with long legs and a perky butt.

In short: She was a goddess!

As time went by, more and more people started arriving, especially the little nuisances and their parents. I looked around and recognized most of the counselors from previous years. All were young pretty girls except Denise. She always dressed in black, Gothic style! I had never been in the mood for such women.

This year Tobias, my best friend and Lisa's older brother, was there again. For the last two years he had a steady girlfriend and preferred to spend his holidays with her. For three months he was single again.

Natalie arrived as one of the last supervisors. She was new this year and seemed a bit boring at first.

On the bus I immediately chose the seat next to Lisa. We were ready to go and when the bus started, she counted twice that everyone was there. Then she distributed the camp passes.

Then she sat down next to me and took a few deep breaths.

We looked at each other briefly and smiled. Since we had known each other for years, there was a comfortable intimacy between us.

Unfortunately, I hadn't seen her for a few weeks because she's studying atmospheric sciences at the University of Innsbruck. To this day I still don't get what it's about, but I didn't want to ask her again.

"How's your studies going? Is there anything new?" I asked.

Lisa told me, beaming with joy.

"I've had a boyfriend for two months."

All of a sudden my good mood was gone, I had to swallow and stuttered slightly.

"Great...uhhh...I'm glad, congratulations."

For years I had hopes that she would fall in love with me. I saw in her the mother of my children, the woman of my life. But she had a boyfriend in Innsbruck.

Stupid Austrians!

So at the first rest stop I looked around for the other supervisors.

I needed a woman to take my mind off things.

Also, I was horny and wanted to fuck.

Stupid Austrians! They had taken all my hopes from Lisa.

Well, then just another supervisor.

But shit, no one was like Lisa.

I went to Tobias who had similar thoughts. He also didn't seem to like any supervisor.

The holiday started anything but great.

The camp was in the middle of a lonely valley in the Swiss mountains. So far, the location has been a big advantage because the supervisors couldn't go out in the evening to meet other boys. They had to be content with us. But now it seemed to be becoming a disadvantage for me.

After crossing the Pfänder tunnel, we reached Switzerland. On the autobahn, it was a two-hour drive towards St. Gallen. Then we reached our destination, the small Walensee in eastern Switzerland. The camp was on the north shore near the small town of Quinten. The lake is 419 m above sea level. M. and has a surface of

24 km^2. In the summer it was ideal for swimming and paddling.

We sniffed the fresh mountain air. It was always fascinating how pure and invigorating the oxygen was. Completely different from what I was used to in Munich.

The 10-man tents that were set up were probably leftovers from the old days of the Swiss army. Ah? Did Switzerland even have an army? No idea! The main thing was that the cheese and chocolate were delicious.

Then our protégés were distributed to the sleeping places. There was a tent for each caregiver.

While the caregivers were full, we were only five male caregivers. We generously offered that one or two more girls could stay with us, but unfortunately they declined this offer.

The first few days were stressful, just exhausting!

You had to constantly watch what the little devils were up to.

Unfortunately, nothing went well with the girls either.

I had to realize that almost all of them were firmly assigned.

Where were the many single women that were always reported in the media? At least not here in Switzerland!

I made two more advances towards Lisa, but she blocked me. On the second try, she warned me that I should accept the fact, otherwise she would see our friendship in jeopardy.

One evening I sat around the campfire with Tobias, and things didn't look any better for him either. We talked about the big day trip the following day, which only needs about half of the caregivers.

We had the day off, so to speak, and imagined what we could do nice things. So we decided on a men's outing in the classic sense: sports and beer. We would first engage in physical activity by paddling along the lake and then drink away our grief over missing women. It was a good plan B.

As the trip began, you could feel the calm descending on the camp. Tobias and I hit another round on the ear.

We started our tour in the most beautiful midday sun. Armed with a boat and paddles, we went to the shore of Lake Walen.

From a safe distance we saw Natalie sunbathing on the jetty. We eyed her from a safe distance. She didn't necessarily look ugly, it was more like boring. This was also underlined by her unflattering clothing: She was wearing a baggy, gray T-shirt and red, knee-length shorts. You couldn't even see a hint of breasts on her. Maybe she had a tad too much fat on her ribs? She seemed unsportsmanlike and more like a housewife with two children.

I looked at Tobias and we agreed without words that she was probably the last chance for this camp.

"I'm not sure though, I think she has a boyfriend too."

I thank you for this encouragement.

We approached the jetty and Natalie recognized us.

"Hello, looks like you guys want to go paddling."

I looked briefly at Tobias. How should one reply to such a clever statement? Did she think we'd go skiing by boat and paddles?

I countered succinctly.

"Hello Natalie, we're just going for a walk with the paddles. The little ones also need some exercise."

She looked at me slightly confused. Damn! Since I had probably lost my last chance for sex.

Tobias was a bit more open and friendly.

"Do you want to come along?"

"If that's okay with you?"

"Clear! Get in, otherwise I wouldn't have asked."

After we were in the boat, Natalie also got on board. The paddling tour has already begun.

"Do you have a specific goal?" she asked.

“Yes, I've always wanted to paddle to Chive Island. I've never managed it in years."

"Chive Island?" she asked as if I had screwed her.

"It's really called that," said Tobias, who probably made a more trusting impression on Natalie.

"It's a small island in the middle of the lake," I explained.

"Sounds good."

Natalie sat in front of me and I eyed her again.

I still had certain doubts. But the hope for sex was stronger. The tour was otherwise rather quiet. We arrived at the small island of chives, carried the boat out of shore, took out the blankets and made ourselves comfortable.

We talked, asked her questions and tried to loosen her up a bit. But she answered rather taciturnly and reservedly. So we changed the topic and talked about the young people in the camp and what the little nuisances had done. We sensed that this topic made her a little more talkative.

A little later I gave Tobias a sign with my eyes that I wanted to bathe. We both got up almost at the same time.

"Enough chatter, let's go swimming."

Natalie looked slightly startled.

"I don't have a swimsuit with me!"

"That's a good thing, because neither do we."

Her gaze still looked uncertain. I tried to convince her.

"Hey, we're all grown ups. I promise not to look away from you."

I stripped completely naked and quickly jumped into the water. Tobias followed me and called out to Natalie, "Come on, it's gorgeous."

"Okay, if you have to."

We eyed her happily as she fussed. She undressed, covering her breasts and crotch with her hands while quickly running into the water. Unfortunately we couldn't see much of her body.

Was she just inhibited?

Was her body embarrassing for her?

Certainly, she couldn't hold a candle to Lisa. But we felt her eyeing us. Did she have a boyfriend? Hopefully not.

We wrestled in the water and tried to involve them. So we often jumped up out of the water, we also touched her. She joked along.

After we had had enough of the cool water, we went outside again. Natalie seemed a little bit more relaxed. Luckily I had brought an extra towel so I could offer her one. We tried to study her while she dried herself. She then wrapped herself in the towel.

"I'm thirsty. Toby, give us something from your backpack," I called out and winked at Tobias. He took a six-pack of beer cans out of his backpack and offered one to Natalie as well.

"I don't think the little one can handle something like that," I countered and seemed to have touched her sensitive nerve.

She defied. "Bah! Give me the part!"

We toasted together. Natalie tried to open the can in a totally cool way and took a deep sip right away. Her facial expressions spoke volumes, she probably didn't like beer. She literally choked it down. But she wanted to look casual and took another sip. When the can was half empty, she was already a little tipsy.

She got funny and giggled around. I look at Tobias, we nodded to each other.

I challenged Natalie.

"I bet you can't swallow the rest of the can in one gulp!"

"Ha, that'll...we'll see."

She started. In fact, she emptied the beer. Now she was slurring and swaying a little. I gave Tobias a sign with my eyes that he should put the beer away.

"See, I'm not...uhh...small."

"No. You're pretty grown up," Tobias replied.

Again we made eye contact and tried to gesture the next steps. So I let my eyes wander to her breasts. I pretended to lose my balance and pulled on her towel, which fell to the floor. She bent down to pick up the towel while we stared pretty straight at her bare breasts.

"Don't stare, you pigs. Haven't you ever seen a naked woman?"

"Yes, of course we have. But right now it's only you. And we can have a look, right?" Tobias answered.

Natalie picked up the towel again and wanted to use it to cover her breasts.

"You are lechers, yes. So! Enough looking."

I tugged at her towel again.

"Oh, come on. Let's see!"

"Nope..."

Now I blinked at Tobias and planned another attack. We gently pulled the towel and her hands away. At first we still felt some resistance, but after the most important body parts were free, she no longer resisted.

She slurred a little more.

I wasn't sure about her situation anymore at that moment. She didn't seem as insecure as she did at first, you could already feel the pride in her. The pride of once hanging out on the beach with two handsome guys who were interested in her. In my mind, I applied rule number one when dealing with questions: Praise! So I tried to appreciate her body.

"The two breasts are really pretty!"

I winked at Tobias again. Almost simultaneously we started rubbing her breasts. At the same time, she lost all shyness and probably let herself fall due to the effects of the alcohol. We felt how lust and desire slowly arose in her.

She protested only slightly.

"Hey, what are you doing?"

"Nothing you don't like," I countered, taking her breast into my mouth. I let my tongue dance over her stiff nipple.

"Ooooooh! Oooh! What are you doing to me?"

I felt her getting really horny and pushed her to the floor. Tobias ran his hand down his thighs. After a moment she voluntarily opened her legs. Tobias reached his goal. He played in her pubic triangle and felt her wetness.

Slowly he pushed a finger into her column.

Natalie groaned. Tobias showed me through his wet fingers how wet and aroused she already was.

"Fine, lick it!" I ordered him.

Tobias knelt before her shame. Natalie opened her thighs further to accommodate his head. As soon as he put his tongue on, she moaned loudly. Luckily there was nobody around who could hear it. Apparently the touch was already too much for her. She cringed slightly.

I took care of her breasts, sucked and licked her nipples.

"Do you like that, Natalie?"

"Yeah, yeah!"

"Have you been licked many times?"

"Nooo, first time"

"Are you still a virgin?"

"Nooo, I've already..."

She was so horny and drunk. We could have asked her about anything. But I preferred to reveal our plans.

"Fine, because afterwards we're going to fuck you both, okay?"

"Yesssssssssssssssssssssssssssssssssssss sssssssssss together

Tobias did a good job. He had a very quick tongue. I devoted myself to her breasts.

Suddenly, I felt a tremor spread through her body.

"Yeah, yeah, good, go on, yeah, I cooooom!"

Then it really trembled. She screamed her orgasm out loud.

"Oh, that was good, so good," she moaned after she'd calmed down a bit.

Meanwhile, our cocks were really hard. To be on the safe side, we opened another can of beer and offered it to her. She drank from it greedily. Then we took the can from her hand and flattened it on the blanket. Tobias crawled between her legs, spread her thighs and pushed his hard penis into her column without big words.

"Oh, it's nice and tight!" he gasped.

The anticipation boiled inside me, but I still had to wait. Natalie acknowledged almost every thrust with a groan.

"Yes, yes, yes, deeper," she demanded.

"Do you like my cock?" he asked.

"Yes, that's good, push it in nice and deep!"

"Am I fucking you good?"

"Yeah, you're great."

"Well, you're good to fuck too. That's the way it should be."

"Then do me right. Yes exactly."

Sometimes Tobias talked too much during sex. But I didn't want to complain, she played along, that's the main thing.

As I knelt by the two of them, I accidentally discovered a video camera that had fallen out of Toby's backpack. I turned it on and filmed the two having sex. Who knows what you might do with it later. Like a reminder. Or to change her mind in the next camp, if there are only taken women there again. Tobias had a good grip on her, he rammed her like a rabbit.

Then the two kissed briefly. Toby got even faster, fucking her two or three more times, then he cummed. As soon as he pumped his sperm into her vagina, he jumped up and took the camera from me. He now filmed Natalie up close, lying on the blanket with her thighs open. I heard the camera zoom.

Now he interviewed her.

"Did you just get licked and fucked?"

"Yes, I am"

"Did you like it?"

"Yeah, it was super awesome."

"You're cheating on your boyfriend right now, aren't you?"

"Yes I do. But as horny as you just banged me, he'll soon be my ex-boyfriend."

"You're a pretty hot bitch."

"Thank you, do what you can."

"Do you want Ben to fuck you now?"

"Yes, please."

"Then say it."

"Please, Ben, fuck me."

You could feel her alcohol level. Because such things are rarely said soberly. But at the latest this little interview brought clarity.

She had a boyfriend, but apparently it wasn't a happy relationship. Anyway, I was asked to fuck her, so I didn't want to refuse her gentlemanly request.

I looked at her light brown triangle of pubic hair, knelt between her spread thighs and rubbed my glans through her crack.

I slowly pushed my penis into her pleasure cave.

Tobias had not exaggerated, her vagina was really very tight. It felt like I was deflowering her. Natalie inhaled and exhaled frantically. She seemed to hurt slightly as I entered her with my penis. Tobias is not badly equipped, but mine is a bit bigger. I slowly slid further into her gorge, pulled him out again and pushed myself deeper again.

"Am I hurting you?"

"No, fuck me."

I didn't let myself be told a request like that twice. Tobias tried a few close-ups with the camera and conducted another interview.

"Does he fuck you good?"

"Yeah!"

"Does he have a longer tail than your ex-boyfriend."

"And wiiii!"

"How is it for you, Ben?"

"Great, a really horny bitch. We're going to have a lot of fun with it."

Luckily Tobias limited himself to the few questions this time. Any more would have been annoying.

I slid in and out of her faster now, thrusting deeper and deeper. I'm probably also touching areas in her that had never been touched before. I could feel her pelvis pressing against me with every thrust. Sweat was already pouring down our bare skin. Then it twitched violently in her pussy.

She screamed so loud it hurt my ear canal.

But the convulsions also helped me climax. We gasped and moaned, looked into each other's eyes, then kissed deeply and deeply. With a huge explosion I pumped my sperm into her uterus. I felt her vaginal muscles vibrate violently from my spurts of semen. It felt great. Natalie was a super fuck toy!

Then I rolled off her slender body. It took us a few minutes to regain consciousness while Tobias took a few more close-ups of her.

Natalie was still totally excited. "Wow, that was something."

"That was great. Are you always this good or is it just us?" I asked her.

"To you. Just the two of you!"

We drank another round of beers and thus kept their level high.

"How about a little dessert?" asked Tobias.

"What do you have to offer?"

"You can put my cock in your mouth."

"Okay, sounds delicious."

I took the camera and filmed the two. Natalie looked a little hesitant. She took his penis and started licking it with her tongue. You could literally see that she hadn't done it that often before.

But Tobias motivated her with more compliments.

"Wow, that's really good. I've had worse blow jobs."

I saw her trying hard to do well. Sexually she was still pretty green behind the ears. You could probably make a real bitch out of her.

"Oh keep it up. Great. Oh yeah. Take it deep inside", he asked her to continue. And she did that too. Now Tobias took the lead. He took hold of her head and determined the rhythm.

"Yes, yes, oh, that's good. I'm about to cum in the bitch's mouth!"

His legs began to tremble, he moaned uncontrollably and pounded his member into her warm mouth. His phallus pulsated, the first splashes landed right in her throat. After she had swallowed everything, he let her go, Natalie collapsed, breathing heavily. She wiped her mouth. Anyway, she seemed to like it.

"You're really not bad as a wind player!"

"Phew, so that's how bubbles go. Not that bad."

I handed the camera to Tobias and stood in front of her with my cock.

"If you like it that much, then go ahead."

"What about me?" she asked expectantly. "I want to have those horny feelings again."

"Okay, then Route 69!"

I lay on my back and pushed her over me. Then I felt her tongue on my glans. At the same time, I began to nibble on her pubic hair with my lips.

She finally managed to take my glans completely in her mouth. She licked her tongue while rubbing her teeth over my sensitive skin.

It felt great.

In the meantime I had found my way through her intimate hair and pushed my tongue into her column. I pushed her in as deep as I could. Why didn't I have a foot tongue? I would be the lick god!

Alas, I was only a mortal man, but besides my tongue I had one finger! A task occurred to me.

There was an untouched entrance just above my nose.

Exciting!

I briefly pushed my index finger into her vagina to moisten it sufficiently. Then

I massaged over her wrinkled anus. Her sphincter spasmed and twitched at my touch. Cool!

As my lips sought her clit, my index finger massaged her anus. I pushed but couldn't get in as she clenched her ass.

Then my lips found her clit. I sucked her pleasure pearl over my tongue and gently nibbled on her. She seemed to like this!

She spat out my penis and screamed loudly. At that moment she relaxed her sphincter. I took advantage of this immediately and slid my finger into her gut.

Suddenly her screams stopped.

She didn't seem to like the fact that my index finger was scanning her intestinal walls. I bit her clit quickly, seeming to distract her from my finger as she started screaming again.

Or did I bite too hard?

Regardless, I sucked and nibbled until she calmed down.

Tobias came in front of her face with the camera.

"Like what Ben is doing?"

"He shoved a finger up my ass!"

"Yes, I know, I filmed it. Do you like that?"

"No, tell him to stick that finger up his own ass."

"He doesn't listen to me."

"What can I do to make him stop it?"

"You should keep sucking his cock, once he has an orgasm your body loses interest."

"Good idea."

She immediately put her mouth over my penis again.

I had found the secret switch to perfect oral sex!

The harder and deeper I pushed my finger into her gut, the more lustfully she sucked my cock.

I could control the beat, rhythm and speed of her blowing activity with my finger in her anus.

Was this the switch I had always wanted in a woman?

Was it hidden on the inner walls of her intestines?

Would I be awarded the Nobel Prize for this groundbreaking discovery?

Anyway, I fucked her anus faster and faster.

At the same time I felt my sperm leaving my testicles and looking for the way to freedom.

Then everything in me exploded.

I reached a sensational climax and pumped my sperm down her throat. She swallowed and swallowed, but couldn't make it all. I could see strands of sperm hanging from the corners of her mouth.

After I had my orgasm her body became really uninteresting. I pulled my finger out of her ass and gave her a hard smack on her buttocks and shoved her aside.

Then we lay on the blanket for a long time, completely exhausted.

We jumped naked into the lake again and cooled off.

Natalie seemed overjoyed.

After a while, hunger drove us back to camp.

In the following days we often used the opportunity to fuck with Natalie. She became greedy and insatiable.

In the moonlight it was really romantic. And when the opportunity arose, we also wandered through the woods during the day. She usually knelt down somehow and we fucked her from behind.

When we got back to Munich, we went our separate ways.

A little later, Lisa, Tobias' sister, called me. She told me that she broke up with her boyfriend and wanted to meet me.

Lisa! My Goddess! My love.

Who was Natalie again?

4

THE WINDOW TO HAPPINESS!

Okay, this might sound strange, but at twenty-two I still live in the attic of my parents' house.

All of my friends at that age already had their own apartment or a steady girlfriend.

That was my second problem.

I didn't have a girlfriend!

I've been single for five years now. I also had no affairs or short-term sexual adventures. The only eroticism in my life was given to me by my right hand.

It wasn't my appearance. I was a handsome guy, with dark brown hair, green eyes, and a slim, athletic body.

It was Chloé!

She's my best friend Tim's younger sister and lives right next door. I fell in love with Chloé five years ago. Since that time, I have not been able to approach, speak to, or take out any other woman. I only thought of Chloé; morning, day and night. In my dreams and in reality.

I could see straight into her room from my skylight. So I stood in front of the window in the morning, day and night hoping to get a glimpse of the love of my life. As long as Chloé lived across the street, I would never move out of my parents' house, even if I was eighty.

As a result, I didn't find time to continue my studies or go out with friends. The window didn't allow it, I couldn't leave the pane of glass alone.

My parents and friends now had serious doubts about my mental health. Maybe they were right. Wasn't love a form of insanity?

Sometimes Chloé would even see me standing by the window and wave to me.

At such a moment my heart stopped.

When it was dark I could watch my friend's sister in her room without being noticed. She had a slender, athletic build and long blond hair, most of which she wore in a ponytail.

One evening I didn't manage to get into my room until a little after 11pm. I was watching football with my father in the living room. It was the Champions League game between Bayern and Arsenal. Unfortunately, I was only able to watch Sky at my parents'. My mood wasn't the best because Bayern also lost 2-0. This was my only passion besides Chloé, by the way; Bayern Munich.

For that alone, some would attest to my insanity.

But anyway, I came to my room after the game. My first way was of course to the window. I noticed that the light was still on in Chloé's room.

She was lying completely naked on her bed!

There was no doubt what she was doing!

She masturbated!

The sight took my breath away. I stopped dead in my tracks and watched as she was about to fuck herself with two fingers of her right hand. With the index finger and thumb of her left hand she kneaded, squeezed and pulled at her hard nipple on her right breast.

I immediately felt a tingling between my legs. A mixture of love and lust arose in my body. My penis got hard!

As I watched her, I massaged my cock in the same rhythm as she penetrated herself with her fingers.

We were one, in love, in spirit, in soul and in jerk off speed. At least I hoped so.

Suddenly she turned her head and looked straight at me!

She looked me in the eyes without stopping fingering herself.

could she see me

I was standing in the dark.

But I could feel her gaze entering my brain through my eyes and finding its way into my heart.

Involuntarily I took a step back. But it was already too late, because Chloé briefly raised a hand and waved at me.

Now I saw it. I left the stairwell light on so she could see my build in the window.

I raised my hand in embarrassment and waved back. Then I stepped from the window and quickly closed the curtains.

Damn, she had actually caught me cocking!

Of course that was incredibly embarrassing! But on the other hand it was her own fault, after all she could have drawn her curtains!

To calm myself, I went into the kitchen, poured myself a wheat beer and took a long sip.

The sight of you had made me totally horny!

Was she still masturbating?

She had probably drawn the curtains by now.

But I was curious.

I went back to my attic room, turned off the light, stepped behind the curtain and pushed it aside a little.

Much to my surprise, Chloé still hadn't closed her curtains and was still lying on her bed, masturbating hard.

She didn't seem too bothered that I could watch her jerk off. So she probably wasn't a prude.

Meanwhile, she massaged her clitoris with quick back and forth movements.

Just as I was pulling down my pants, cradling my hard cock, she suddenly rose, got on her knees, grabbed a large pillow from the edge of the bed and tucked it between her legs.

Then she actually did it!

She began rubbing her vagina against the pillow with wide back and forth movements of her hips.

She fucked the pillow!

"Oh my god!" I groaned.

Another touch would have been enough and my sperm would have slapped against the window pane.

Watching Chloé's wild ride on her pillow, I hastily stripped down my pants and jerked my cock.

A little later my body trembled and I pumped my seed down onto the parquet floor. I came very hard and could hardly stand up, my knees were shaking. As my orgasm slowly subsided, I staggered to the bathroom. When I got there, I first drank cold water, washed my hands and my hot face. After a shower, I rushed back to my window.

But Chloé had meanwhile closed the shutters, so there was nothing more interesting to see. She had probably reached her climax long ago as well.

The next evening I quickly went to the supermarket. I had just paid and was pushing my shopping cart out of the store when suddenly Chloé came towards me.

I expected her to complain about my cocking yesterday, but she walked towards me with a friendly smile.

"Hello, Harry," she spoke in her wonderful voice. "How are you?"

"Uhh... hello Chloé, thanks... uhh I'm fine and about yesterday, I'm really sorry! I didn't want to watch you...uhhh, I was about to close the curtains and..." I stuttered in embarrassment.

"...and then you just couldn't look away, right?" she grinned teasingly at me, which threw me off even more.

"Oh, no, no! I then... I wanted...", I stammered a bit in panic.

"All right! You do not have to apologize! I could have drawn the curtains! But I don't mind that you watched me. In fact, it actually turned me on quite a bit, to be honest! If you know what I mean," she explained.

"Uhh... no... not really."

"I like it when you watch me from your skylight. It turns me on, I guess I'm a little exhibitionist!"

She smiled at me.

"Oh, okay, if that's the case, then I'm relieved. I thought I disturbed you."

"No, just the opposite! I thought it was cool!"

She grinned cheekily in my face.

"Unfortunately, I have to go now! See you soon," I stammered.

"Yes, hopefully see you soon," said Chloé in a friendly farewell.

When I got home I had to sort my thoughts.

Chloé an exhibitionist?

You didn't mind that I was secretly watching you?

The later it got, the longer I stood at my window and waited for her. But everything was still dark.

Just as I was slowly giving up hope, I suddenly noticed a light in her room.

I quickly turned off the TV and the light. I hid behind the curtain and stared spellbound.

There was nothing to be seen for a few agonizing minutes, but then she suddenly stepped into the room. She had wrapped a large bath towel around her body and was drying her wet hair. Apparently she had just showered.

To my delight, it wasn't long before she opened the bath towel and draped it over the back of a chair. Now she was standing naked in her room, still drying her long, blond hair.

Her beautiful, slender body was tanned and in good shape. She had beautiful perky breasts with large nipples. Her tight ass was easy to bite into. Her privates was covered by a triangle of blond pubic hair.

In wise foresight, I had only put on a loose shirt. My penis dangled freely between my legs.

Chloé had since taken to applying lotion to her arms and legs. Then her hands wandered further over her slender stomach up to her breasts. Again she dribbled some lotion into her hand and rubbed it slowly and happily with both hands over her beautiful breasts. Creaming became caressing and finally tender kneading.

She obviously enjoyed it. Even from this distance I thought I could tell that her nipples were hard and swollen. Just like my penis!

Chloé put one leg on the edge of the bed, spread her legs, dribbled lotion into her hand and actually began to cream her vagina, or rather to massage it with relish.

I suddenly noticed that she was looking in my direction!

She couldn't possibly see me. The light was off and I was hiding behind the curtain.

Why was she still looking at my window?

Could she sense that I'm watching her?

So I made a spontaneous decision!

I rushed to the coffee table and switched on the lamp. Then I went back to the window and pulled the curtain aside.

After a moment's hesitation, I walked shirtless in front of the window and looked down at Chloé

Our eyes met!

I raised my hand briefly and waved at her. Without stopping massaging her blond-haired vulva with her right hand, she raised her left hand and waved back.

My heart was pounding!

As I watched her masturbate, I cupped my hard cock and gently pulled back the foreskin. My glans throbbed and longed for more touches.

She finally lay on her back on her bed, her privates pointing directly in my direction. Then she bent her legs, spread her thighs and grinned conspiratorially at me. I had a perfect view of her slightly parted labia.

She put both hands to the left and right of her column and presented her wet column to me! A hot shiver ran through my body at this incredibly hot sight!

From the angle and height of my window frame, I was certain that Chloé could only see me up to about my navel, so she could only guess what I was doing to my cock.

But I didn't want to deprive her of that!

It would have been unfair. So I got a chair, put it in front of the window and climbed up.

I was now a good 50 cm higher, so I was sure that she could clearly see my stiff penis.

She confirmed that immediately by giving me a thumbs up.

I started jerking off my hard studs again as she stroked up and down her cunt and teased her nipples with her other hand.

When she finally slowly pushed two fingers into her horny hole, I had to remove my hand from my member for a moment, otherwise I would have come. My penis jerked and bobbed up and down without me touching it.

I couldn't believe how aroused I was not only to watch Chloé masturbate, but to know that she was watching me too!

I was always horny!

Suddenly she sat up, turned around and stretched out her tight buttocks towards me. With her left hand she first stroked her buttocks. Finally, she massaged her clearly visible rosette with her middle finger and slowly pierced her sphincter.

The sight of her fingering her wet vagina and her horny anus at the same time was finally too much for me.

An unbelievable orgasm shot through my body, so that I could hardly stay in the chair.

She had turned her head to the side so that she could see exactly how my sperm spurted out of my cock and shot against the glass pane of the window. Thrust after thrust I emptied my penis.

At this sight, Chloé also reached her climax.

She bucked briefly, then fell flat on the bed, shaking with a few violent convulsions. For a while she lay on her stomach, stunned.

After a brief respite, she sat up, turned back to me, looked me straight in the eyes, and licked her finger.

I blew her a kiss, which she returned.

My heart skipped a beat.

I felt this gesture as if she had actually kissed me.

My Chloe! My Goddess!

We said goodbye with a short greeting.

The next evening the doorbell rings.

My parents were at a Helene Fischer concert, so I had to open the door myself. I pulled on a pair of jogging pants and rushed downstairs. After opening the front door, I almost fell backwards against the wardrobe.

Before me stood Chloé!

She smiled at me while my mouth dropped and I was unable to greet her.

"I wanted to say thank you for yesterday! I thought it was great that you watched me. My climax became much more intense under your gaze," she explained.

I still couldn't make a sound.

"May I look at your window? I'd like to see your angle of view of my room."

I nodded my head in agreement, still unable to make human sounds. She sure seemed to think I was a brainless monkey.

Smiling, she walked past me and climbed the stairs to my attic room. I slammed the front door and followed her.

When I reached my room, she was already standing in front of my window and looked at her own realm.

"You have a good view of my bed," she stated. Her fingers searched for the remains of my sperm on the glass pane.

What should I say?

Hi? Earth to Harry. Please send suitable words!

"I hope you masturbate more for me and let me watch," she said, licking her finger with the bits of sperm that were still stuck to the glass pane.

Those should have been my words!

"Uhh... yes... gladly," I stammered.

What nonsense was that? Earth to Harry, please send a reasonably articulated sentence and not mindless babble.

She turned and looked me straight in the eyes.

My knees threatened to buckle.

"Did you like that I watched you do it?" she probed.

"Yes, very much so," I ground out as a first attempt at a reasonable sentence. "Didn't it bother you, Chloé?"

"But on the contrary. I was amazed at how much it turned me on," she replied.

"Sounds very confusing to me," I said, more likely to say something and break the silence.

"We are hermaphrodites."

"Please what?"

"Intersexed."

I must have rarely looked stupid because she laughed heartily.

"I mean, we're a mixture of exhibitionist and voyeur. A hermaphrodite, we like to watch each other, but we also need this feeling of being observed."

"I haven't looked at it that way, Chloé."

"But it's true, isn't it?"

"Hm."

"Do you like to watch me?"

"There is nothing in this world that I wish for more."

She smiled softly at me, her eyes sparkling.

"Did you enjoy my watching you?"

"There is nothing more beautiful in this world than feeling your eyes on my body."

She smiled again.

"The same thing happened to me! So we're hybrids," she grinned at that statement.

There was a longer pause during which she looked at me closely. My cheeks turned a soft blush.

"Well, if we like to watch each other, how about we just do it right in front of each other. Shorten the distance."

"Uh... what do you mean?"

"We could just do it right now! Let's undress and watch each other do it!"

"You want to masturbate in front of me?" I stammered.

"Yes, if I can watch you too. You know we're hybrids! Watch and be watched."

I did not know what to say. My body pumped blood into my abdomen, my penis stiffened and pressed against the fabric of my sweatpants.

"He would like it," she said with a smirk on her face, looking at the bulge in my pants.

"You're right, Chloé," I finally admitted. "I couldn't imagine anything nicer."

"Great! It's definitely going to be awesome!" she exclaimed enthusiastically. "How should we do it? Will you sit on the armchair and I on your bed?"

"Uhh... yes, please," I stuttered again.

While I was still in the process of pushing the armchair in front of my bed, she quickly took off her clothes. Before I knew it, she was sitting completely naked on my bed with her legs spread. For a brief moment I was speechless.

"You've seen all of me for years, haven't you?"

"Uh... yeah..."

"How long have you been watching me?"

"Since 1792 days."

"You know that exactly?"

"Yes, I will never forget a single day."

She gave me a look that made my heart clench, my pulse quickened, and put moisture on my forehead.

"You're cute, Harry. Undress yourself!"

I quickly took off my shirt and pushed down my sweatpants including panties. My penis had reached a degree of hardness that was already like a weapon.

She leaned forward and eyed him at close range. She seemed to be scanning every vein, skin fold, and pubic hair. I stood perfectly still, like a Greek statue being admired by tourists.

"You are beautiful," she said, smiling, raising her head and meeting my eyes.

"Uh...thanks," I stammered again like a little kid being handed a pacifier.

"So is your penis, by the way," she added.

She smiled.

I was about to have a heart attack. My blood pressure was probably 220/160, my heart rate was 120.

Did she know what each of her words did to my body?

She leaned back, drew her legs up and placed her feet on the edge of the bed. I had a direct view of her wide open labia and could clearly see that her crack was already glistening with moisture.

"How do you like my vagina?" she asked while she put both hands on her thigh and pulled her outer labia apart with one finger of each hand, so that her dark red slit opened even more.

"You were created by Michelangelo before you returned to Olympus, right?"

"You are sweet."

She started stroking her wet cunt up and down with her right hand. With the middle finger of her left hand she massaged her clitoris, which had protruded from the skin fold.

"I want to watch you too," she said decisively.

I carefully wrapped my hand around my hard cock. Any movement would have triggered my instant orgasm, I was already that horny.

"Oh yeah! You have an amazing cock! I really like your penis. Why didn't you show it to me sooner," she moaned while shoving two of her fingers deep into her vagina.

"Watch me fuck myself for you and do it to you too!" she gasped while penetrating herself with her fingers faster and faster.

I, too, began to work on my cock. As if under hypnosis, I couldn't take my eyes off her fingers. I heard the loud smacking of her fingers, saw the wetness dripping out of her vagina.

"Oh yeah! That's so cool. Jerk off your hard cock, do it for me!" she moaned loudly, pulling her fingers out of her crack, putting them both in her mouth and sucking on them.

"Oh god I'm so wet! I love watching you," she wailed in lust while dipping her fingers into her dripping hole again.

"Does it turn you on when I lick my juice off my finger?" she asked while panting while licking her fingers for the second time.

"Oh yeah and how!" I gasped as well. "I love everything you do. A goddess can't make mistakes."

"You are sweet."

She slid her index and middle fingers into her cleft again with relish, pulled them out and licked them with the tip of her tongue.

"Yes! Lick her clean!" I gasped.

"You make me so horny! I'm about to cum!" she moaned louder and louder as she finger fucked herself faster and faster, rubbing her clit with rapid movements.

A heavy scent of sex and lust hung in the air.

After a while, Chloé was finally ready!

"Oh God! I'm coming! Ohh jaaaa!" she practically screamed. With a last deep "ohhhhhh" she reared up. Her body went through several wild convulsions as a gush of her cum dripped onto my bed.

I watched her spellbound as she slammed into a really intense orgasm right in front of me that barely seemed to stop.

Then it came to me too.

I reached my climax pumping my cum in massive spurts onto the floor, across the bed, even hitting her thigh.

It took quite a while for our bodies to calm down.

"Oh wow! That was really a great orgasm!"

With a cheeky grin, she added, "Did you like it Harry?"

"Oh god, yes and how!"

She pulled her labia apart again.

"My pussy is still dripping!"

She rubbed her wet hole with three fingers, spreading her juice all over her blonde pubic hair.

"Come to me, Harry," she said tenderly.

I got up and sat next to her on the bed. She pulled me down and pressed her lips to my mouth.

It was the first time in my life that I was allowed to kiss a goddess!

Our lips parted and our tongues began a loving play. Every touch created a flash in my body.

She gently stroked my stomach with her fingernails and realized that just from the kiss my penis was sticking out of my body again in full hardness.

"You're stiff again, Harry."

"This is what happens when a goddess gets involved with a human."

"You are sweet."

She rolled over me, grabbed my penis and guided it between her labia. Slowly, without breaking eye contact, she lowered herself. I penetrated her pleasure cave inch by inch.

She put her hands on my chest and let her pelvis rotate slowly. She seemed to like this position.

She soon forgot how ecstatic she had just arrived. Back and forth, up and down, back and forth she spun her bottom and almost heard the angels singing again, she was so aroused by this game.

I massaged her soft back with my fingers.

She shivered from tiptoe to nipple as she felt my cock inside her, directing it the way it felt best with sleepwalking certainty. When I cupped her firm breasts and gently pinched her swollen nipples, she was crushed.

Unlike the previous one, this orgasm slowly surged in, ebbing back a little only to return more intensely. Softly whimpering, she experienced shivers after shivers and just when she thought it was over, she shook again. She had never felt anything like this in her entire life.

I stayed completely still inside her and enjoyed the twitching of her body. Having just hosed down, I was still enduring.

A sweet languor took possession of all her limbs. She felt a slight, not uncomfortable tug in her vagina. Instinctively she knew that after this Mount Everest of highlights she would not come again. She lifted her pelvis to free herself from me, crawled to the side and stretched her bottom towards me.

"Please fuck me from behind, my darling," she breathed.

Treasure? Did she really say darling?

I couldn't think about it any longer because my cock wanted to go back into her warm cave.

So I knelt behind her and willingly let her guide me. She grabbed my cock through her legs and guided it gently but firmly to her crack. As my head dipped into her cave, I thrust my hips forward. With an intense thrust, I penetrated her with my entire length.

I grabbed her hips and pushed her hard. She clawed her hands into the bedding and tried to return my thrusts with equal intensity. I gripped tighter, rotated my hips, and varied the pace. I slowly retreated to her gate, only to strike again.

Our bodies smashed together on my bed like two great beasts mating with a roar.

I came shortly after!

I pumped my sperm into her vagina with huge spurts. Chloé started shaking all over, rolling her eyes and screaming out her orgasm.

We had our climax at the same time and sank into a sea of lights, stars and fireworks.

At that moment, we felt an invisible band wrap around our bodies. Our souls seemed to merge.

"I love you Harry."

"I've loved you for 1792 days," I replied.

"You are sweet."

She pulled me towards her and we melted into a kiss that was never allowed to end.

5

RAINY CONCEPT!

"I'm here, finally!"

Those were my thoughts when I found this lake. The way was pure torture. The forest aisle was totally sandy and with the bike it was more than just exhausting. In addition, the entire area was very hilly. And since it was neither signposted nor visible in any way, I drove right past it. I had to fight my way through the bushes for the last few meters. After finding the lake, at least I was compensated. It was a natural idyll that is rarely known.

And it was in the middle of nowhere, in the deepest and loneliest part of Bavaria. The special thing was that this romantic place, unlike all the other lakes in the area, had no name.

I dropped into the sand and enjoyed the solitude. It was a place without hassle.

I wanted to swim, but unfortunately I had left my bathing suit at home. So I only went in up to my ankles. I saw small fish passing me which was a good sign in lakes like this. As dusk slowly fell, I made my way back.

But the very next day I wanted to go back to the lake, this time with my bathing suit. Even if the way was exhausting, it was good for the condition.

As if by chance I found my place again, which was not so easy with the dense bushes. Then I dropped onto the sand and dozed for half an hour. Then I wanted to go into the water. I had already put on the bikini at home. I took off my skirt and shirt.

Standing in water up to my knees, my inner urge for freedom won out. I stripped completely naked and threw my bikini on the ceiling. I think there is nothing nicer than feeling the cool water of a forest lake on your bare skin.

I caught some giggles from afar, a sign I wasn't alone.

Should I bring the bikini back?

No, I went through with it.

But I stopped for a moment and took a 360° look around. There were indeed some people here, but they were very spread out. One could almost say that everyone had their own bay here. And most of the people here seemed to be naked as well. If I still remember the outdoor pools, where they all scratch around the pool like brood hens, it's just freedom. I also saw that the lake stretched quite a bit along. Far more than I could see from my small space.

On the way back, a swimmer passed me quite quickly. He greeted me. For a moment I thought it was a come-on, but the guy really just wanted to be friendly, otherwise he barely noticed me. When I got back to my bay, I felt absolutely no need to cover myself. I felt free. it was my lake

For me it was a completely different attitude to life than on the nudist beaches with their double standards. There, where guys roam the ranks, constantly staring at women's breasts in order to secretly jerk off later.

Since that day I have made a pilgrimage to this lake almost every day. Once I met an old woman who, like me, was turning from the forest path to the lake. We got talking and she told me a flashback. She was now seventy years old and knew the lake from her youth. She discovered that here she could escape from textile society. A few years later came the hippies and some '68ers. They sat down and sang songs. It didn't bother her, but she was afraid that the lake could become a crowd puller. Since then she has called the lake 'Hippie Lake'. Fortunately, interest in the lake has also waned. And she still liked coming here, although her husband was suspicious and would think she was cheating on him, but on the other hand he also liked her complete tan.

That's how I got into conversations with a few people. Most tend to be athletic. Because if you can't cycle or jog, or at least hike like the old woman, you'll never come here. And for a Mallorca vacationer who is in Germany to save up money, there will certainly be too little action here. Especially since there is no road or parking lot here. Here are the people who tick differently. Close to nature, sporty with a preference for nudity.

The lake still seemed to have some meaning for hippies, so I occasionally heard loud 70s music.

I also happened to overhear a couple having sex and no one was itchy. I watched the two of them pampering themselves for a few minutes, but in the end it was nothing special!

An impressive experience was three young men arriving in a canoe and paddling across the lake. Anyone who can carry such a canoe for kilometers through the forest no longer needs weight training. I was cheeky once and asked the guys if I could go with them, no problem. It was a great feeling when you, as a woman, sit at the front with the wind blowing in your face and three muscular guys sitting behind you and swinging the paddles. And all naked. But I didn't get the feeling that they were staring now, even if we were scrutinizing each other a bit. But that was only with the eyes, without ulterior motives.

The summer was coming to an end. According to the weather report, it should be the last really hot day. And again I was drawn to the lake, meanwhile I didn't even take my bikini with me anymore.

While it was unbearable in Munich, the climate at the lake was quite pleasant. So I peeled off my clothes and went to cool down. As I swam my laps, another swimmer crossed me. I looked into his eyes for a moment, then we greeted each other. As he swam past, my subconscious said, 'You know this guy'. The voice, the face. But I still wasn't sure.

When I got back to the beach, I pondered for a while. And while I was dozing, the penny dropped. It was Patrick, my older brother's best friend. He was two years older and my unrequited childhood love. Unfortunately he had moved to Vienna to study. At first I was heartbroken, but as we all know, time heals all wounds.

What was Patrick doing in Munich again?

But, was it really him?

He looked so different, only his bright brown eyes still felt warm in my stomach.

How should I find out?

Just asking would have been stupid.

'He who doesn't dare, doesn't win' was my formula.

When I saw him gliding gracefully through the lake, I spontaneously dived into the water. I made my way so that we crossed each other.

We smiled at each other again.

'Now or never', I thought and followed him.

It was quite a challenge, but for a short time I succeeded. When he turned and came towards me again, I gathered my courage.

"You're not Patrick by any chance?"

He stopped swimming and looked at me.

"Yes. How do you know me?"

I looked at him and had no more doubts. He was it!

"Cool. Guess what!"

I saw his brain convolutions working. Then he smiled.

"You're Sarah, Julian's little sister, right?"

I nodded and smiled at him.

"What a surprise. It really is you."

I splash him with water.

We swam to shore, straight to its bay. When the water got shallow we ran. And when the water was at step height, I had to take a quick look at him. His lean, muscular body made my pulse quicken. His slightly curved penis created warmth in my sex.

The memories suddenly came back.

How in love I had been with him!

We lay down in the sand, close together and looked at the clouds. We felt we had a lot to tell each other. What we did back then and what drew us to this lake. He found nature and tranquility particularly important here.

Then I couldn't hold back any longer. There was a topic that had accompanied me for years and had not been clarified until today.

"Do you remember my birthday wish?"

"What do you mean?" he asked curiously.

"My fourteenth birthday. You sat in the garden with my brother and asked me what I wanted as a present. Do you remember my answer?"

"Yes, of course, I'll never forget that," he replied. "You wished for a kiss."

"Why didn't you kiss me? It was my birthday wish!"

"I know I'm sorry. You looked so young and fragile. Your brother laughed and I was confused. I thought this was fun, hidden camera or something."

"I was really disappointed."

"I am sorry."

"It's not my birthday today," I said in a calm voice. "But you can fulfill my wish from back then. You owe me a kiss!"

"Okay, but it's my present."

"What do you mean?" I asked in surprise.

"I dictated the manner of the kiss, okay?"

"Of course, your gift, your rules."

"Yes, but it should at least be a French kiss."

He had to laugh.

"You're still the Sarah I knew!"

At that moment, I wasn't really aware that the term 'French kiss' could be interpreted differently. Here my mouth was indeed faster than my brain. I lay there completely relaxed and without any ulterior motives while he crawled over to me and smiled seductively at me. I expected his lips to approach my mouth to pay the kiss debt.

But I was wrong!

With his gentle hands he grabbed my thighs and spread my thighs. My labia gaped slightly. He knelt between my legs and approached my private parts with his face.

"What are you doing?" I asked, startled.

"My gift, my rules, remember?"

"But aren't you too deep for a kiss?"

"Did I say which lips I would kiss? You have two beautiful wet specimens here too."

"Bunker," I said, grinning at his cheek.

"But I will grant your wish. You get a French kiss, a very wet one at that."

Then I felt his mouth kissing my vagina.

Then it came, the tongue!

He touched my clitoris and I had to moan briefly. But the tongue did not disappear again. Like French kissing, he set her in motion. He circled my clit and labia.

"OK! OK. You have redeemed your debt of honour."

But Patrick didn't think about ending the French kiss!

On the contrary, he used my clit as a counter-tongue to encircle it. I wanted to push him away. But I found myself getting weak, literally.

What situation have I put myself in here?

How do I get out of here unscathed?

But I really didn't think so anymore. To be honest, I just lay in front of him and enjoyed the French kiss. I opened my thighs even further and came towards him a bit. He stroked my stomach with his hands and explored my erogenous zones. But I didn't really get it anymore.

The feelings in my abdomen dominated. I was moaning loudly now. And so slowly I felt my orgasm come.

He seemed to recognize this.

For a moment he stopped the movement of his tongue and remained, but without breaking away from my embarrassment.

When he felt that the wave had subsided again, he continued at twice the pace. From now on he gave no mercy, constantly licking, kissing and sucking on my private parts.

Then I came!

My orgasm rolled over me.

I saw colorful stars, felt my blood pressure somersaults. My eyes went black for a moment while I felt such wonderful feelings as never before in my life.

My abdomen was shaking and shaking so badly that he had trouble holding the kiss. As the trembling subsided, he pulled his lips away from my vagina. He lifted his head, smiled at me and licked his mouth with the tip of his tongue. I was still a little taken aback by his side and enjoyed the fading of my orgasmic waves.

"Oh, I'm really sorry. I didn't know you twitched like that when you kissed."

For a moment I was speechless. It was me who usually had the pointed tongue.

"Shall I tell you something, you scoundrel? You don't look like you're sorry at all. Otherwise you might have asked if I'm still okay?"

"I did, the body language with you worked really well."

At this point his tongue was just sharper.

"Well, now you're speechless. You could actually, well, how should I put it, you could also give me something for my birthday. Quid pro quo, you know what I mean?"

"As? Would you like a French kiss too?"

"Of course, what man wouldn't?"

"I don't kiss every man!"

"Then prove to me that I'm not just any man to you."

"You're nasty!"

"No, cool! Look how hard my penis is. He would be very happy about a French kiss."

We both laughed.

I had to go inside myself again.

Did I really want to do this?

should i do it

I was at a loss for a moment.

In the end I thought, well, I'll do it, I'll do him a favor.

I moved into a better position and grabbed his aroused phallus.

"He feels good," I breathed, really impressed by the size and thickness of his cock.

"Your hand feels good too, I'm curious if your tongue is similarly comfortable."

"You are naughty!"

"You're shy because I can't feel anything on my penis yet."

I bit him very gently on the glans.

"Ouch. You are confusing something. The tongue is the soft thing in the middle of your mouth."

"Thanks, I'm already aware of the anatomy!"

I licked the glans once, stopped what I was doing and looked at him cheekily.

"What is? Why don't you continue?" he asked, raising his eyebrow.

"Oh, suddenly I don't really feel like it anymore."

I emphasized that so teasingly that the intention of the words was quite clear: I wanted to play with him a bit more!

"Why then?"

"Then I'll explain it to you. Before a woman puts a man's penis in her mouth, she wants to hear that she's something special. So think of a compliment and I'll do my best."

He smiled. His eyes were beautiful.

“Sarah, even then you were the most beautiful girl I had ever seen. You are the girls' Mona Lisa, unique and beautiful. The little dream princess has become a really attractive and very erotic woman."

His words took my pleasure for a moment. My heart clenched as if an invisible hand was squeezing. My pulse quickened, my blood pressure increased.

They were the nicest compliments I had ever heard from a man. And those words came from Patrick, my childhood sweetheart. I had to be careful not to cry.

"You... uh... that was beautiful," I stammered. "You really deserve a French kiss now."

I noticed how he was slowly getting fidgety. Another interruption would certainly have resented his penis. But I didn't want to spoil it with his genitals, who knows what else I might need him for.

Full of feeling I licked his hard shaft up and down with the tip of my tongue. I felt how he was very sensitive, especially on the underside. I kissed his scrotum with my lips, playing with his balls. He closed his eyes and let himself fall.

I alternated my hands between his shaft, which I moved back and forth, and his balls.

I encircled his glans with my lips and now let my tongue dance. I often got stuck on the ribbon and played with it. Patrick literally melted away.

As I ran my tongue over the opening, I could clearly hear him gasping for air. I felt myself in control of him and increased the pace. The tongue constantly alternated between the frenulum and the opening, as well as occasionally circling the glans.

In the meantime, Patrick could hardly be held back. I could feel his tight ass trembling beneath me, pushing his cock in and out of my mouth. For a moment I thought about what else I could do for him as a favor, but just then he reached his climax.

I was just in time to pull his penis out of his mouth when he squirted his sperm into the sand as I jerked off.

"Somebody seems to have liked his birthday present."

"I would like to have a birthday every day."

"I also."

They were wonderful moments together. I just felt comfortable around him, had no shame or shyness.

We then went back into the water to cool off; swam a few lengths.

"By the way, I meant what I said before. You've turned out to be a very attractive woman."

"Thanks, you're embarrassing me."

He smiled and took my hand and held it tight as if creating an invisible bond that would bind us together forever. We stayed like that for a few minutes with just a few movements.

When we reached its little cove again, we lay down on the sand. I felt at that very moment that something had arisen between us or had existed for a long time.

We lay on our backs, looked at the sky, didn't speak and enjoyed the physical proximity to one another. Then we got back to talking. Exactly where we lived, what we were doing and what we planned to do in the future.

"Well, let's be honest. Did you actually think about me again after I moved to Vienna?" he asked.

"But already. Very often even. Unlike you, you didn't even recognize me when I spoke to you!"

"What made you so sure it was me anyway?"

"Your eyes."

Now I started to ask him something.

"And what else can you remember from our time then?"

“You were so young, so shy and fragile. I was afraid to talk to you, you always blushed easily."

"I seemed shy to you?"

"You were fourteen or fifteen, so it's normal to be shy, isn't it?"

We smiled at each other, getting closer as if we were poles of a magnet inevitably pulling towards each other.

He ran his hand through my hair and stroked it back. Then he approached with his face until our lips touched and joined in a kiss.

I was exposed to a roller coaster of emotions.

The feelings that I had already overcome came back. The same romantic infatuation. Could it be more?

Or is it just the happy hormones that the sun released in me today? It wasn't quite clear to me yet. And maybe, I thought, by the next day I would hate myself for what I had gotten myself into.

As he kissed me, his fingers caressed my body. He touched my breasts, playing with my nipples until they stuck out hard from my body. Then his fingers danced over my flat stomach and shortly thereafter reached my pubic triangle.

I spread my legs.

He recognized this as an invitation and tenderly rubbed my clitoris.

I was almost dizzy with excitement. Everything was spinning, I seemed to be running out of pleasure.

"I want you, Patrick," I breathed. "But it doesn't work."

"Why?"

"I'm not using birth control, or do you want to hear the stork padding?"

Patrick turned sideways, dug a condom out of his pocket and held it under my nose with a grin.

"Soso, a prepared young man."

I guided his hand straight to my vagina. That was the point of no return. At least morally.

But I wanted to feel him inside me. His finger did a good job and after just a few minutes I felt physically ready.

I slipped the condom over his enormous penis.

Since he was already lying on his back, I was allowed to start with my favorite position: the rider.

I sat on him and played with his cock so that he caressed my labia. But I haven't let him in yet.

I looked into his eyes. His eyes communicated with me. They looked expectant. They told me to finally let him in. I could always be a beast. And so I still moved my abdomen very gently. I had hoped that he would ask me, challenge me, or penetrate me with dominance.

But nothing came except that loving look.

"Do you dare?" I asked teasingly.

His hands were immediately on my butt and he pushed it down. With one hand he briefly positioned his cock. I didn't resist, I wanted to be guided. He did now. And he did well. Bit by bit it slipped into my vagina.

It feels good!

When he was completely inside me, we lingered for a moment. I enjoyed the feeling. We played with the eyes.

"What have you nasty rascal done to me here?" I asked him in an erotic voice. I licked my lips and began very gently with the riding movements.

"I was just helping you. You had such a pleading look like you wanted to be fucked."

"You can read minds."

"It was easy to spot."

Slowly the words were no longer clear, but embedded in audible breathing noises. I felt his cock throbbing.

"Just the way you're going about it. how you want to annoy me It seemed like a game of lust."

"I play?"

"Yes! But is a dangerous game"

"Oh! I love dangerous game."

I bent down to him and gave him a kiss that expressed all my lust and love. Then I started pacing faster, sliding his cock in and out. It feels good. He began to use his hands as well. He stroked my clitoris with one hand and grabbed my breasts with the other. Subconsciously, I realized that he was just touching her for the first time, so late in the act. Men usually grab my tits first.

I had forgotten everything around me.

I didn't care if anyone heard me either. In case of doubt, it didn't matter here. I rode him like there was no tomorrow. And his finger drove me insane.

It was cool, the game of lust.

We got faster. And faster. And I could feel his cock throbbing inside me, twitching. As the semen shot through his trunk into the rubber.

He was panting and breathing quickly and raggedly.

As his climax wore off, he sat back exhausted.

Unfortunately, it wasn't enough for me, but I let myself fall on him first. Patrick had gradually acclimatized again.

"Hey, but the dangerous game isn't over yet!"

"Soso, the sweet little devil wants more."

I demonstratively bit his shoulder.

"Yes! That's what you've got!

"You used to be a shy girl."

“Oh no, no nostalgic please. Go on, show that you're a real man and that you can handle it. Oh no, don't go limp!"

I pulled off the condom and lovingly took care of his penis. Oddly enough, the sperm didn't bother me, on the contrary, I didn't care. It tasted good.

I licked, nibbled, sucked and played with his head.

Since Patrick had already come twice, it took a little longer to make him horny again. But the fight was worth it. I found the most beautiful moment when he slowly straightened up. Where you could see the good, valuable piece filling with blood.

I looked at him dog-eyed and wanted to ask a question, but he seemed to know my thoughts.

"Sorry, but I don't have a second condom with me."

I let go of his cock and looked deep into his eyes.

"But I still want to come," I said, disappointed.

"Then slide it in, it's ready."

“You are aware that this can be a very dangerous game. I don't use contraceptives," I explained.

I started gently scratching his stomach with my fingernails. Sometimes I also pricked him.

"Yes, my sweet, beloved goddess," he said full of feeling. "I am aware of the responsibility and will be careful."

beloved goddess?

Did he feel similar feelings to me?

His half-declaration of love took away all inhibitions from me.

I lay flat on my back, spread my legs and smiled defiantly at him.

He met my gaze and knelt between my thighs. His swollen glans stroked through my thick pubic hair and looked for the entrance to my column.

I felt him slowly slide his penis into my receptive cleft. Full of greed and lust, I enjoyed how I was filled piece by piece by his hard member.

Exactly this is the most exciting moment for me.

I closed my eyes and just wanted to enjoy, to be lazy so to speak and not exert myself.

Patrick did well in his role. He wasn't that fast, not too slow, I was able to keep up with him and relax. Neither of us seemed ready to come anytime soon.

Patrick after two highlights anyway.

A lot of time passed in this position.

A lot of time!

And that's exactly what I needed. At some point I began to feel the first signs of a new peak that was still a long way off.

While I was only breathing intensively up to now, I now began to moan softly. That also turned Patrick on to get a little faster.

Suddenly I felt a drop on my eyelids. Nothing unusual, probably just a drop of sweat from Patrick. Then came the second. And the third. A striking number.

It began to rain!

"Oh, shit," I heard him say. I could feel him trying to pull himself out of the affair, but I wrapped my legs around his back, preventing him from pulling away from me.

"I don't like wimps. Only real men!" I said sternly, giving him the signal to continue shagging me.

Practically the rain didn't matter at first, whether we got wet from sweat or from rain didn't matter. So I also became active in the lower position in the missionary and kept stretching my pelvis towards him. My orgasm was not far away.

He increased the pace. I felt that I would soon be ready.

I moved my hand down and touched my clit. Suddenly the orgasm was there. And how he was there.

I literally screamed. I gasped. I shook myself. I felt it twitch. I especially felt him twitch. I hear him panting. We twitched together. We kissed intensely. We were still breathing quickly. I enjoyed the cock in me for a moment. We cuddled. I had an incredibly good feeling. I was happy.

Unfortunately, reality caught up with us.

Distracted by the rain and my intense orgasm, he forgot to pull his penis out of my vagina in time.

He pumped his sperm into my fertile vagina!

Did he notice?

"I have to get to my things!" I shouted, jumped up and dived into the lake. As I swam to my cove, I felt his sperm trickle out of my crack.

As I feared, my clothes were completely soaked. Only my towel in the backpack was still dry. But anyway, I put on my skirt and wet t-shirt, packed my backpack and pushed my bike through the forest.

Patrick is already waiting for me at the forest aisle.

We faced each other.

"I've wanted to tell you this for years, Sarah. I love you!"

That's when I jumped on him. Like Dino with the Flintstones when Fred came home. He had trouble not falling over. But he mastered that. i kissed him

"I've loved you for as long as I can remember, Patrick."

I literally hugged him and kissed his face, he returned it. We caressed each other forever while the rain completely soaked our bodies. But we didn't feel any of that.

The meeting at the lake is now two years ago.

Luckily our paths didn't diverge again.

We now have an apartment together
and a fourteen-month-old daughter.
The lake and the rain forged our luck.
A love that I hope will last forever.

www.ingramcontent.com/pod-product-compliance
Lightning Source LLC
LaVergne TN
LVHW012054160826
845678LV00014B/2816

* 9 7 9 8 3 5 2 3 9 2 7 5 1 *